MOSBY'S REVIEW FOR THE
CLINICAL COMPETENCY TEST

Small Animal Medicine and Surgery

MOSBY'S REVIEW FOR THE CLINICAL COMPETENCY TEST

Small Animal Medicine and Surgery

Ellen Miller, DVM, MS, Dipl ACVIM
Associate Professor
College of Veterinary Medicine and Biomedical Sciences
Colorado State University
Fort Collins, Colorado;
Diplomate
American College of Veterinary Internal Medicine

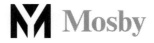

St. Louis Baltimore Boston Carlsbad Chicago Naples New York Philadelphia Portland
London Madrid Mexico City Singapore Sydney Tokyo Toronto Wiesbaden

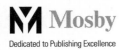

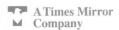

Vice President and Publisher: Don Ladig
Editor: Paul W. Pratt
Senior Developmental Editor: Teri Merchant
Project Manager: Linda McKinley
Production Editor: Rich Barber
Manufacturing Manager: Linda Ierardi

Printed in the United States of America
Composition by Top Graphics
Printing/binding by R.R. Donnelley & Sons

Mosby–Year Book, Inc.
11830 Westline Industrial Drive
St. Louis, Missouri 63146

International Standard Book Number 0-8151-4379-6

97 98 99 00 01 / 9 8 7 6 5 4 3 2 1

CONTRIBUTORS

Ellen N. Behrend, VMD, MS, Dipl ACVIM
Department of Physiology & Pharmacology
College of Veterinary Medicine
Auburn University
Auburn, Alabama;

Thomas H. Boyer, DVM
San Diego, California

Derek P. Burney, DVM, Dipl ACVIM
Houston, Texas

Brian G. Loudis, DVM
Denver, Colorado

CONTENTS

INTRODUCTION

J.L. Rothstein and P.W. Pratt

State and national board examinations have long been surrounded with mystery, misunderstanding, and anxiety. To help candidates prepare for licensure examinations, Mosby has published a series of review volumes. *Mosby's Review for the Clinical Competency Test* is a two-volume work that prepares candidates for the Clinical Competency Test (CCT). *Review Questions & Answers for Veterinary Boards* comprises five volumes to prepare candidates for the National Board Examination (NBE).

Candidates sitting for national and state board examinations will find these review books a valuable resource, as they comprehensively cover all subject areas included on veterinary licensure examinations.

Veterinary students can benefit by using these books as practice tests during courses and also to review material before final examinations as each course is concluded.

Practicing veterinarians will find the books useful for continuing education. Veterinarians moving to a new locale can use them to prepare for licensure examinations in their new state or province. The books also aid preparation for specialty board certification, particularly for certification by the American Board of Veterinary Practitioners (ABVP).

Foreign graduates can use these review books as they prepare for the Education Commission for Foreign Veterinary Graduates (ECFVG) certification examination.

How to Prepare for Licensure Examinations

Develop a Strategy

You can begin your preparations for licensure examinations by developing a study plan and a strategy for taking the tests. Studying the many subjects covered in the examinations is only one element of the strategy. Before you begin studying, determine which tests you will be required to take. State and national jurisdictions often have different licensure requirements. For example, all jurisdictions require the NBE, and all except the District of Columbia and the Virgin Islands require the CCT. Depending on the state(s) you plan to practice in, you may have to pass their state board examinations.

Are You Eligible to Take the Examinations?

Determine if you are now or when you will be eligible to sit for the required examinations. Many states allow junior (third-year) veterinary students to take board examinations. For many students, this is an ideal time to take the national board examinations. At this time, they are heavily involved in classroom study and the information is relatively fresh in their minds. They have also begun their exposure to clinical practice through rotations in the university's veterinary teaching hospital. Additionally, many students favor taking the board examinations at this time because there is relatively little pressure to pass; if they do not pass the first time, they can take the tests again during their senior year.

When and Where Are the Examinations Offered?

Determine the dates, times, and locations of upcoming licensure examinations. Typically, the NBE and CCT are offered together in April and December each year. Not all states administer the tests, and they offer the examinations on various dates. Also, the cost for taking the examinations may vary substantially from one state to the next; knowing this ahead of time might influence your decision on which state examinations to take.

Many candidates delay their initial fact finding until a few weeks before the examinations are offered. Such procrastination is unwise and unnecessarily stressful; it may take several months to obtain all pertinent test information. Don't waste your energy worrying about whether you will be permitted to take the test or if you will be registered on time. Gather this information well ahead of time so you can devote your full energy to studying for and passing the tests.

6 Months Before the Examination

Become Familiar With the Examination Requirements: Obtain test information on the NBE and CCT from the Professional Examination Service (PES, 475 Riverside Drive, NY, NY 10115, telephone 212-870-2724).

Gather specific information on licensure requirements, examination dates, and costs for each state where you would like to gain licensure. Refer to the licensure requirement list at the end of this introduction for general guidelines. For more detailed information, consult the *Directory of Veterinary License Requirements,* available from the American Association of Veterinary State Boards (AAVSB, P.O. Box 1702, Jefferson City, MO 65102, telephone 573-761-9937).

Develop a Master Study Plan: Your plan should include:
- A list of subjects to review and emphasize
- A realistic time frame for review of specific subjects
- A general study schedule
- Resources for studying (materials, study aids, groups, review sessions, etc.)

3 Months Before the Examination

Register for the Examinations: Make final decisions about which examinations to take and then register for those examinations. This process is often more complicated and time-consuming than you might think. Many states only accept certified checks. Some have exacting requirements you must fulfill before they will let you sit for the test. Avoid problems and reduce anxiety by taking care of these details well ahead of time.

Reevaluate Your Study Plan: Develop a fairly rigid study schedule for the last few months of study before the examination, allotting sufficient study time for both the CCT and NBE. Begin to focus more on review sessions with other people and study groups. It is easy to become bored with studying during the several-month preparation period. Diversifying your study techniques helps maintain your interest level and improves retention of subject information.

Maintain a Positive Frame of Mind: Many candidates are overwhelmed by the immense amount of material they must review. The period of preparation for licensure examinations can be stressful; however, you can redirect the stress to your benefit. Develop a positive attitude and consider the examinations a challenge.

In preparing for the examinations, you will learn many useful things and will review information learned earlier but forgotten. Ultimately, all of the information reviewed during your preparations will serve you well, during the remainder of your veterinary education and in the practice of veterinary medicine. By taking a positive approach and beginning your preparations early, you can reduce your level of stress and do a better job preparing for the examination.

Reviewing for the CCT

Structure of the CCT

The Clinical Competency Test (CCT) was developed to assess a candidate's ability to manage clinical cases, such as those encountered in practice. The CCT is a 4-hour examination given in conjunction with the NBE, in April and

December of each year. Each year, over 3000 candidates take the CCT and NBE.

The CCT currently consists of 14 case management problems, with approximately 1000 answer options. Each case problem has 50 to 75 questions, in step-by-step progression, on patient history, diagnosis, treatment, and prevention or control. There are four problems on small animals (dogs, cats), one on exotic species, six problems on food animals (cattle, pigs, sheep, goats, poultry), three problems on horses, and at least one problem on food safety, public health, or epidemiology. Students in a curriculum weighted toward one species area (small animals versus large animals) and graduates now practicing exclusively in small animals or large animals should direct their study efforts toward areas with which they are less familiar.

Each case problem begins with an opening scene that outlines the clinical situation (patient characteristics, presenting signs, history, etc.). The questions for each problem are then presented in stepwise fashion, as in actual clinical practice. The questions are usually grouped in sections pertaining to patient history, physical examination, diagnosis, treatment, and prevention or control. The questions are printed in standard black ink in the left-hand column of the page. The answer choices are printed in latent-image ("invisible") ink in the right-hand column. Candidates choose answer options using a marker pen to reveal answers printed in latent-image ink. As the problem progresses, each answer choice revealed with the marker pen provides feedback on that decision or action, and guides candidates in making further choices in managing the case.

Each CCT problem is designed around an "optimal pathway" of case management. The optimal pathway comprises only the answer choices associated with the correct diagnosis and proper case management. Candidates are penalized for failing to select choices in the optimal pathway and for selecting choices that do not lead to resolution of the case.

CCT Scoring

In veterinary practice, not every choice in managing a case is clearly indicated or clearly contraindicated. Some actions are neutral (i.e., they do not help resolve the case, but neither do they harm the patient or impede case management). Scoring of the CCT attempts to reflect this real-life situation. Some answer choices are "clearly indicated" (essential in resolving the case), some are "clearly contraindicated" (must be avoided in managing the case), and some are "neutral" (neither indicated nor contraindicated).

The answer choices in the CCT are "weighted" with regard to point value. Answer choices in the early sections of a problem, such as on history taking, tend to be worth fewer points (positively or negatively) than those in later sections, such as on treatment. Your score on the CCT is based on the aggregate of correct choices (points added) and incorrect choices (points deducted).

A "perfect score" on the CCT is 800, with candidates achieving an average score of approximately 500. The passing score varies among licensing jurisdictions. Some assign a "pass" or "fail" score. Some use a "criterion-referenced" passing score based on the scores achieved by the entire population of candidates sitting for the CCT at that time. Other states use a "locally derived" passing score. In jurisdictions requiring both the NBE and CCT, your CCT and NBE scores are combined to determine if you pass or fail the licensure examinations.

The Practice CCT

Carefully read the CCT information booklet and take the practice CCT available from the Professional Examination Service (PES). This material provides insight into the subject areas emphasized on the examination, shows you how the CCT is structured, and allows you to practice using the marker pen to highlight answer options.

CCT Test-Taking Strategy

Performing well on the CCT involves more than knowing medical and surgical facts and procedures. You must understand how the test is scored and how to avoid penalizing yourself when making your answer choices. On the CCT, *you are penalized for incorrect answers.* Points are allotted for correct answers but deducted for incorrect answers; some answers are "neutral," so points are neither gained nor lost. Once you reveal an answer with the marking pen, it cannot be changed and is considered as part of your total score. The strategy discussed below focuses on selecting the greatest number of correct answers, rather than avoiding incorrect answers.

Read the Opening Scene Carefully and Develop a Short List of Differential Diagnoses: The structure of some of the case problems can lead you toward an incorrect line of reasoning. Proceed carefully and don't jump to conclusions by locking onto a specific diagnosis early in the problem. Consider all of the possibilities on your list of differential diagnoses, not just the first one that comes into your head.

Understand the Scoring Procedure: Let's assume each case problem has 50 questions, worth a total of 100 possible points. Questions on the history and physical examination, for example, are worth 5 points each, diagnostic tests are worth 10 points each, and diagnosis and treatment are worth 15 to 20 points each. As you proceed through the problem, the point value increases, but you are answering fewer questions per section. Remember, you earn points for each correct answer, lose points for each incorrect answer, and neither earn nor lose points for "neutral" answers.

If You Have Little Idea of the Correct Diagnosis, Do Not Guess: Many candidates believe that, to pass the CCT, they must answer every question in a case problem. This is an erroneous assumption and can lead to failure. To the contrary, it may be to your advantage to answer some but not all of the questions in some sections of the case problem, and answer only the questions about which you are reasonably confident. Rather than trying to answer every question correctly, focus on answering most of the questions correctly and avoiding guesses that could heavily penalize you. Consider this technique as you take the practice CCT supplied by PES.

The CCT tends to have more low-value questions on history, physical examination, and diagnostic tests, and fewer high-value on treatment and control. As you finish the diagnostic test section, perhaps you will have accrued 50 or 60 points. If you are fairly sure of the correct diagnosis and proper treatment, you can proceed with confidence. Incorrectly guessing at a diagnosis leads to selecting incorrect answer choices throughout the remainder of the problem. This will likely cost you 25 to 40 points, leaving you with a score of only 10 to 35 points for that problem.

Consider Diseases Emphasized in Past Examinations: Certain diseases appear to receive more attention on the CCT than others. Although the emphasis may change from time to time, common diseases are almost sure to be covered in the CCT. While it is important to have a broad-based study plan, make sure you know the basics first. It is more important to have a firm grasp of major diseases than it is to know a limited amount about every disease ever reported.

Following is a list of diseases or conditions more likely to appear on the CCT:
- *Dogs and cats:* renal failure, diabetic ketoacidosis, hyperadrenocorticism, hypoadrenocorticism, hyperthyroidism, hypothyroidism, gastric dilatation-volvulus, pyometra, osteochondritis dissecans, ununited anconeal process, fractured medial coronoid process, patellar luxation, cruciate ligament rupture, hip dysplasia, abdominal neoplasia, neurological disorders, scabies, demodicosis, ringworm, allergic dermatitis, autoimmune disease, glaucoma, retinal disorders, cystitis, urolithiasis, congestive heart failure, feline leukemia virus infection, feline immunodeficiency virus infection, feline infectious peritonitis, toxoplasmosis, kennel cough, and parvovirus infection.
- *Cattle:* traumatic reticuloperitonitis, vagal indigestion, abomasal ulcers, abomasal displacement, bloat, Johne's disease, foot and mouth disease, bluetongue, rinderpest, malignant catarrhal fever, bovine virus diarrhea, lead poisoning, listeriosis, thromboembolic meningoencephalitis, grass tetany, polioencephalo-malacia, pseudorabies, hypovitaminosis A, urea poisoning, postparturient paresis, bovine respiratory syncytial virus infection, infectious bovine rhinotracheitis, parainfluenza virus-3 infection, pasteurellosis, *Micropolyspora faeni* infection, pulmonary emphysema and edema, tracheal edema, calf scours, blackleg, tetanus, botulism, malignant edema, enterotoxemia, anthrax, anaplasmosis, tuberculosis, pyelonephritis, lymphosarcoma, ketosis, urolithiasis, vesicular stomatitis, mastitis, actinobacillosis, actinomycosis, leptospirosis, infectious keratoconjunctivitis, anaplasmosis, necrotic pododermatitis, winter dysentery, white muscle disease, trichomoniasis, brucellosis, warfarin toxicity, and lightning stroke.
- *Horses:* fractures (miscellaneous), navicular disease, laminitis, thrush, pedal osteitis, osselets, ringbone, bucked shins, splints, curb, sole abscess, colic, reproductive disorders, neonatal isoerythrolysis, equine viral arteritis, equine herpesvirus-1 infection, influenza, equine infectious anemia, encephalomyelitis (EEE, WEE), strangles, heaves, guttural pouch mycosis, choke, laryngeal hemiplegia, Potomac horse fever, babesiosis, joint and navel ill, tetanus, botulism, recurrent uveitis, foal diarrhea, and nutrition.
- *Pigs:* clostridial enteritis, colibacillosis, proliferative enteritis, salmonellosis, swine dysentery, cryptosporid-iosis, coccidiosis, whipworm infection, epidemic diarrhea, rotaviral enteritis, transmissible gastroenteritis, actinobacillosis, pasteurellosis, atrophic rhinitis, mycoplasmal pneumonia, Glasser's disease, swine influ-enza, pseudorabies, porcine reproductive and respiratory syndrome, erysipelas, *Streptococcus suis* type-2 infection, group-E streptococcal infection, thromboembolic meningoencephalitis, salt poisoning, heat stroke,

greasy pig disease, sarcoptic mange, parvovirus infection, leptospirosis, hog cholera, swine vesicular disease, African swine fever, eperythrozoonosis, iron deficiency, brucellosis, mulberry heart disease, osteochondritis dissecans, sanitation, ventilation, and farrowing management.
- *Sheep and goats:* foot and mouth disease, bluetongue, dermatophilosis, lead poisoning, and orf.
- *Exotic animals and poultry:* distemper in ferrets, insulinoma in ferrets, hypovitaminosis C in guinea pigs, wet tail in hamsters, snuffles in rabbits, psittacine beak and feather syndrome, Pacheco's disease in birds, and Newcastle disease in poultry.

Note: The list above is for general guidance only and is certainly not all inclusive; other conditions not listed above may also be included on the CCT.

Use Your Head and Don't Panic: Many candidates do well on the CCT by using logic. They may not know the specifics of a disease, but they know appropriate clinical procedures and can deduce most of the correct answers. Don't panic if you encounter a problem concerning a condition that is absolutely baffling. Occasionally these problems are included to assess your ability to work through a clinical case in which the diagnosis is unknown. Approach these puzzlers as with any other case problem. Use sound clinical judgment to deduce the answers; don't guess if you are unsure of an answer.

Resources for Study

Following are some resources to help you prepare for licensure examinations:

Review Books and Other Written Materials

- General texts on specific subject areas (e.g., internal medicine, surgery, etc.).
- Board review books (e.g., *Review Questions & Answers for Veterinary Boards, National Veterinary Medical Series*)
- Practice CCT and NBE (from PES)
- Old licensure examinations (unofficial and in circulation among students)
- Class notes (from veterinary school courses or continuing education courses)
- Review articles in veterinary journals (e.g., from *Compendium on Continuing Education for the Practicing Veterinarian, Veterinary Medicine*)

Review With Other Candidates, Review Courses

- Study with a group of other candidates
- Study with a partner
- Review sessions hosted by faculty
- Board examination review courses (e.g., course offered by Dr. Richard Stobaeus, Animal Care Clinic and Conference Center, Brunswick, Georgia)

Included at the end of this introduction are the licensure requirements for various jurisdictions, and the addresses of veterinary licensure boards.

Conclusion

Careful preparation is the key to passing the licensure examinations. Review the subject matter and know the licensing requirements of the states in which you want to practice. Become familiar with the structure of the CCT and how the CCT is scored. Take the practice CCT to learn how best to select answers. These preparations will reduce your anxiety and let you concentrate on passing the examinations.

What happens if you do not pass the licensure examinations on your first attempt? Certainly, not everybody passes on the first try. Try to determine the areas in which you fared poorly and concentrate on these areas when studying for the next examination. The key is to develop a good strategy as outlined above. With a positive attitude and a well-considered study plan, you should do well.

We hope these review books will serve as a foundation for your continued success.

Examination Requirements for Various Jurisdictions

Jurisdiction	CCT/NBE Offered?	State Board Exam Required?	Junior Test Scores Accepted?	Call for More Information
ALABAMA	YES	YES	YES	205-353-3544
ALASKA	YES	YES	YES	907-465-5470
ALBERTA	YES	YES	NO	403-489-5007
ARIZONA	YES	YES	YES	602-542-3095
ARKANSAS	YES	YES	YES	501-224-2836
BRITISH COLUMBIA	YES	YES	NO	604-266-3441
CALIFORNIA	YES	YES	NO	916-263-2610
COLORADO	YES	NO	NO	970-894-7755
CONNECTICUT	YES	NO	YES	860-509-7560
DELAWARE	YES	NO	NO	302-739-4522
DISTRICT OF COLUMBIA	NO	YES	YES	202-727-7450
FLORIDA	YES	YES	NO	904-487-1820
GEORGIA	YES	YES	NO	404-656-3912
HAWAII	YES	YES	NO	808-586-2694
IDAHO	NO	YES	YES	208-332-8588
ILLINOIS	YES	NO	NO	217-782-1663
INDIANA	YES	YES	YES	317-233-4407
IOWA	YES	YES	NO	515-281-5305
KANSAS	YES	YES	YES	913-456-8781
KENTUCKY	YES	YES	YES	502-564-3296
LOUISIANA	YES	YES	NO	504-342-2176
MAINE	NO	YES	YES	207-624-8603
MANITOBA	YES	YES	NO	204-945-7651
MARYLAND	NO	YES	YES	410-841-5862
MASSACHUSETTS	YES	YES	YES	617-727-3080
MICHIGAN	YES	NO	YES	517-335-0918
MINNESOTA	YES	YES	YES	612-642-0597
MISSISSIPPI	YES	YES	YES	601-324-9380
MISSOURI	YES	YES	YES	314-751-0031
MONTANA	NO	YES	YES	406-444-5436
NEBRASKA	NO	YES	YES	402-471-2115
NEVADA	NO	YES	NO	702-322-9422
NEW BRUNSWICK	YES	YES	NO	506-851-7654
NEW HAMPSHIRE	NO	NO	YES	603-271-3706
NEW JERSEY	NO	YES	NO	201-504-6500
NEW MEXICO	NO	YES	YES	505-841-9112
NEW YORK	YES	NO	NO	518-474-3867
NORTH CAROLINA	YES	YES	YES	919-733-7689
NORTH DAKOTA	NO	YES	YES	701-328-2655
NOVA SCOTIA	YES	YES	NO	902-865-1876
OHIO	YES	NO	YES	614-644-5281
OKLAHOMA	YES	YES	YES	405-843-0843
ONTARIO	YES	YES	YES	519-824-5600
OREGON	YES	YES	YES	503-731-4051
PENNSYLVANIA	YES	YES	YES	717-783-1389
PUERTO RICO	YES	YES	NO	809-725-7904
QUEBEC	YES	YES	NO	514-774-1427
RHODE ISLAND	NO	YES	NO	401-277-2827
SASKATCHEWAN	YES	YES	NO	306-955-7862
SOUTH CAROLINA	NO	YES	NO	803-734-4176
SOUTH DAKOTA	NO	YES	YES	605-773-3321

Examination Requirements for Various Jurisdictions—cont'd

Jurisdiction	CCT/NBE Offered?	State Board Exam Required?	Junior Test Scores Accepted?	Call For More Information
TENNESSEE	YES	YES	YES	615-367-6282
TEXAS	YES	YES	YES	512-305-7555
UTAH	NO	YES	YES	801-530-6628
VERMONT	NO	YES	NO	802-828-2875
VIRGIN ISLANDS	YES	YES	NO	809-774-0117
VIRGINIA	YES	YES	YES	804-662-9915
WASHINGTON	YES	YES	NO	360-586-6350
WEST VIRGINIA	NO	YES	YES	304-558-2016
WISCONSIN	YES	YES	YES	608-266-0483
WYOMING	NO	YES	YES	307-777-7515

Notes

This information was compiled in 1966. Check with the appropriate state licensing agency for The NBE is required by all jurisdictions except the District of Columbia and the Virgin Islands.
The NBE and CCT are offered in April and December every year.
Passing scores are the same in all jurisdictions. Some state and provincial examinations cover only jurisprudence issues. Check with individual licensing boards.

Veterinary Licensing Boards in the United States and Canada

Alabama
Executive Director
Board of Veterinary Medical
 Examiners
PO Box 1968
Decatur, Alabama 35602

Alaska
Division of Occupational Licensing
Department of Commerce &
 Economic Development
PO Box 110806
Juneau, Alaska 99881

Arizona
Executive Director
Veterinary Medical Examining
 Board
Room 230
1400 W. Washington
Phoenix, Arizona 85007

Arkansas
Executive Secretary
Arkansas Veterinary Medical
 Examining Board
1 Natural Resources Drive
Little Rock, Arkansas 72215

California
Executive Officer
Veterinary Medical Board
Suite 6
1420 Howe Ave.
Sacramento, California 95825

Colorado
Program Administrator
Colorado Veterinary Medical
 Examining Board
Suite 1310
1560 Broadway
Denver, Colorado 80202

Connecticut
Connecticut Board of Veterinary
 Medicine
150 Washington St.
Hartford, Connecticut 06106

Delaware
Board of Veterinary Medicine
PO Box 1401
Dover, Delaware 19903

District of Columbia
District of Columbia Board of
 Veterinary Examiners
Room 913
614 H St. NW
Washington, DC 20001

Florida
Executive Director
Florida Board of Veterinary Medicine
1940 N. Monroe St.
Tallahassee, Florida 32399

Georgia
Executive Director
State Examining Boards
166 Pryor St. SW
Atlanta, Georgia 30303

Hawaii
Executive Officer
Board of Veterinary Examiners
Box 3469
Honolulu, Hawaii 96801

Idaho
Board of Veterinary Medicine
PO Box 7249
Boise, Idaho 83707

Illinois
Veterinary Board Liaison
Department of Professional
 Regulation
320 W. Washington
Springfield, Illinois 62786

Indiana
Board Director
Health Professions Bureau
Room 041
402 W. Washington St.
Indianapolis, Indiana 46204

Iowa
Secretary
Iowa Board of Veterinary Medicine
2nd Floor
Wallace Building
Des Moines, Iowa 50319

Kansas
Executive Director
Kansas Board of Veterinary
 Examiners
10475 Purple Sage Rd.
Wamego, Kansas 66547

Kentucky
Kentucky Board of Veterinary
 Examiners
PO Box 456
Frankfort, Kentucky 40602

Louisiana
Executive Director
Board of Veterinary Medical
 Examiners
Suite 604
200 Lafayette St.
Baton Rouge, Louisiana 70801

Maine
Division of Licensing and
 Enforcement
Department of Professional and
 Financial Regulation
State House Station 35
Augusta, Maine 04333

Maryland
President
State Board of Veterinary Medical
 Examiners
50 Truman Parkway
Annapolis, Maryland 21401

Massachusetts
Executive Secretary
Board of Registration in Veterinary
 Medicine
Room 1516
100 Cambridge St.
Boston, Massachusetts 02202

Michigan
Licensing Administrator
Michigan State Board of Veterinary
 Medicine
Department of Commerce
PO Box 30018
Lansing, Michigan 48909

Minnesota
Executive Director
Board of Veterinary Medicine
Room 102
2700 University Ave. West
St. Paul, Minnesota 55114

Mississippi
Executive Secretary
Mississippi Board of Veterinary
    Medicine
209 S. Lafayette St.
Starkville, Mississippi 39759

Missouri
Executive Director
Missouri Veterinary Medical Board
PO Box 633
Jefferson City, Missouri 65102

Montana
Board of Veterinary Medicine
Department of Commerce
Lower Level, Arcade Building
111 N. Last Chance Gulch
Helena, Montana 59620

Nebraska
Section Administrator
Division of Professional and
    Occupational Licensure
Department of Health
PO Box 95007
Lincoln, Nebraska 68509

Nevada
Nevada State Board of Veterinary
    Medical Examiners
Suite 246
1005 Terminal Way
Reno, Nevada 89502

New Hampshire
Secretary-Treasurer
New Hampshire Board of Veterinary
    Medicine
PO Box 2042
Concord, New Hampshire 03302

New Jersey
New Jersey State Board of
    Veterinary Medical Examiners
PO Box 45020
Newark, New Jersey 07101

New Mexico
Executive Director
New Mexico Board of Veterinary
    Examiners
Suite 400-C
1650 University Blvd. NE
Albuquerque, New Mexico 87102

New York
Executive Officer
New York State Board for Veterinary
    Medicine
Room 3043
Cultural Education Center
Albany, New York 12230

North Carolina
Executive Director
North Carolina Veterinary Medical
    Board
PO Box 12587
Raleigh, North Carolina 27605

North Dakota
North Dakota Veterinary Medical
    Examining Board
c/o Board of Animal Health
1st Floor, J Wing
600 East Boulevard Ave.
Bismarck, North Dakota 58505

Ohio
Executive Secretary
Ohio Veterinary Medical Licensing
    Board
16th Floor
77 S. High St.
Columbus, Ohio 43266

Oklahoma
Executive Officer
Board of Veterinary Medical
    Examiners
PO Box 54556
Oklahoma City, Oklahoma 73154

Oregon
Executive Secretary
Veterinary Medical Examining
    Board
Suite 407
800 N.E. Oregon St.
Portland, Oregon 97232

Pennsylvania
Chair
Pennsylvania State Board of
    Veterinary Medicine
PO Box 2649
Harrisburg, Pennsylvania 17105

Rhode Island
Administrator
Division of Professional Regulation
Department of Health
Room 104
3 Capitol Hill
Providence, Rhode Island 02908

South Carolina
Administrator
Board of Veterinary Medical
    Examiners
PO Box 11293
Columbia, South Carolina 29211

South Dakota
Executive Secretary
Board of Veterinary Medical
    Examiners
411 S. Fort St.
Pierre, South Dakota 57501

Tennessee
Administrator
Board of Veterinary Medical
    Examiners
283 Plus Park Blvd.
Nashville, Tennessee 37217

Texas
Executive Director
Texas State Board of Veterinary
    Medical Examiners
Suite 2-330
333 Guadalupe
Austin, Texas 78701

Utah
Bureau Manager
Division of Occupational and
    Professional Licensing
PO Box 45805
Salt Lake City, Utah 84145

Vermont
State Veterinary Board
Office of Professional Regulations
109 State St.
Montpelier, Vermont 05609

Virginia
Virginia Board of Veterinary
   Medicine
4th Floor
6606 W. Broad St.
Richmond, Virginia 23230

Washington
Program Manager
Veterinary Board of Governors
1300 S.E. Quince
Olympia, Washington 98504

West Virginia
Executive Secretary
Board of Veterinary Medicine
1900 Kanawha Blvd. East
Charleston, West Virginia 25305

Wisconsin
Bureau Director
Wisconsin Veterinary Examining
   Board
PO Box 8935
Madison, Wisconsin 53708

Wyoming
Secretary-Treasurer
Wyoming Board of Veterinary
   Medicine
4th Floor, 2020 Carey Ave.
Cheyenne, Wyoming 82002

Canada

Candidates interested in practicing in
Canadian provinces should
contact those licensing boards at
the following addresses:

Alberta
Secretary-Treasurer
Board of Veterinary Medical
   Examiners
#100
8615 149th St.
Edmonton, Alberta T5R 1B3

British Columbia
Board of Veterinary Medical
   Examiners
Suite 155
1200 W. 73rd Ave.
Vancouver, British Columbia V6P
   6G5

Manitoba
Registrar
Veterinary Medical Board
Agricultural Services Complex
545 University Crescent
Winnipeg, Manitoba R3T 5S6

New Brunswick
Registrar
Board of Veterinary Medical
   Examiners
PO Box 1065
Moncton, New Brunswick E1C 8P2

Nova Scotia
Executive Officer
Board of Veterinary Medical
   Examiners
15 Cobe Quid Rd.
Lower Sackville, Nova Scotia B4C
   2M9

Ontario
Registrar
College of Veterinarians
2106 Gordan St.
Guelph, Ontario N1L 1G6

Quebec
General Director and Secretary
Board of Veterinary Medical
   Examiners
Suite 200
795 Avenue du Palais
St. Hyacinthe, Quebec J2S 5C6

Saskatchewan
Registrar
Board of Veterinary Medical
   Examiners
Unit 104
112 Research Dr.
Saskatoon, Saskatchewan S7N 3R3

HOW TO USE THIS CCT REVIEW BOOK

Each case problem begins with an opening scene that outlines the clinical situation (patient characteristics, presenting signs, history, etc.). The questions for each problem are presented in stepwise fashion, as in actual clinical practice. The questions are grouped in sections pertaining to patient history, physical examination, diagnosis, treatment, and prevention or control.

Answer Choices

In the CCT, the questions are printed in black ink in the left-hand column of the page. The answer choices are printed in latent-image ("invisible") ink in the right-hand column. Candidates choose answer options using a marker pen to reveal answers printed in latent-image ink. In this book, the answer choices are printed in black ink next to each question. As you progress through the problem, use a piece of paper to obscure the answer choices, and reveal each answer choice in turn. To help you keep score, circle each answer you selected. In the Appendix you will find normal physiological values and normal blood values for the case studies.

Weight of Answer Choices

As in the CCT, the answer choices in this book are "weighted" with regard to point value. Some answer choices are "clearly indicated" (essential in resolving the case), some are "clearly contraindicated" (must be avoided in managing the case), and some are "neutral" (neither indicated nor contraindicated). Answer choices that are clearly indicated are signified by a "+." Choices that are clearly contraindicated are signified by a "−." Choices that are neither indicated nor contraindicated are signified by a "0."

Assessing Your Performance

These simulated case problems are designed to give you practice in taking the CCT and to point out weak areas in your subject knowledge and case-management abilities. You can generally assess your performance on each case problem by counting the total number of positive (+), negative (−), and netural (0) responses. A preponderance of positive answers, with some neutrals and few negatives, indicates good case-management skills and adequate knowledge of the disease presented in that problem. Conversely, a preponderance of negative answers, with some neutrals and few positives, indicates that you should review the disease presented in that problem.

Opening Scene:

The owner of a Cockatiel presents the bird to you at your clinic. The owner found the bird today at the bottom of the cage. The bird has also stopped eating. In the exam room it is breathing heavily, the feathers are fluffed up, and it is not very responsive to the activities occurring around it. She says it appears to be straining to go to the bathroom.

Go to Section A

Section A:

What questions would you like to ask the owner? *(Choose only the questions you believe relevant to managing the case at this point.)*

1. How many birds are in the house?	1. "It's the only bird I have."
2. When did you first notice that the bird was ill?	2. "Just today."
3. Has there been any change in its behavior?	3. "It has been tearing up newspaper and huddling in the corner of the cage for the past couple of days."
4. What is the diet?	4. "It eats seeds mostly and some frozen corn and peas."
5. Has there been any change in the diet?	5. "No."
6. What is the sex of the bird?	6. "I don't know."
7. How often do you clean the cage?	7. "Once a week. I give fresh food daily."
8. Has there been any change in the stool?	8. "Just today. They are greener and bigger than normal."
9. Has the bird been to a veterinarian before?	9. "No."
10. How long have you owned the bird?	10. "Since it was a baby, 3 years ago."
11. Where did you get the bird?	11. "At a pet store."
12. Is the bird exposed to any other birds?	12. "She gets her nails trimmed at the pet store once a month."
13. Have there been any past medical problems?	13. "No."

Go to Section B

Section B:

Which physical examination procedures would you like to perform at this time? *(Choose only the procedures you believe relevant to managing the case at this point.)*

14. Measure the rectal temperature.

15. Do not perform a physical exam due to the condition of the bird. Place it in a cage and check it in the morning.

16. Weigh the bird.

17. Check the pupils.

18. Examine the oral cavity.

19. Palpate the crop.

20. Palpate the breast muscle.

21. Auscultate the heart and lungs.

22. Use an otoscope to examine the ears.

23. Palpate the abdomen.

24. Examine the stool in the cage.

25. Perform a digital rectal exam.

---

14. The bird starts bleeding from the rectum.

15. The bird is found dead in the bottom of the cage. End of problem.

16. The bird weighs 108 grams.

17. The pupils are normal.

18. The mouth is pink and dry with no discharge.

19. The crop is empty.

20. The keel is palpable but not prominent. The bird is in good flesh.

21. The heart rate is 220 beats per minute; the respiration rate is 60 and clear.

22. The ears are small and the otoscope hurts the bird.

23. There is a firm, smooth oval mass about 1.5 cm diameter occupying the entire caudal abdomen.

24. The stools are loose and voluminous. The feces are slightly green, but the urates are white.

25. The bird starts to bleed from the vent.

Go to Section C

Section C:

Based on the information you have at this time, what diagnostic tests would you like to perform? *(Choose only the procedures you believe relevant to managing the case at this point.)*

26. Draw 2 cc of blood for a complete blood count.

27. Draw 0.10 cc of blood for a complete blood count.

---

26. The bird collapses and dies. End of problem.

27. The complete blood count results show the following:
white cell count = 4500/mm^3
PCV = 46%
Total protein = 3.5 g/dl
Heterophils = 80%
Lymphocytes = 20%
Slight polychromasia

28. Draw 1 cc of blood for a complete blood count and serum chemistries.

28. The complete blood count results show the following:
white cell count = 4500/mm³
PCV = 46%
Total protein = 3.5 g/dl
Heterophils = 80%
Lymphocytes = 20%
Slight polychromasia
Serum chemistries are as follows:
AST = 85 U/L
Calcium = 6.5 mg/dl
Total protein = 3.5 g/dl
Uric acid = 5.0 mg/dl
Glucose = 225 mg/dl

29. Perform a bacteriologic culture of the stool.

29. The results will be available in 4 days.

30. Take a whole body radiograph of the bird.

30. The radiograph revealed normal heart and lungs and a smooth, ovoid mass with a distinct radiopaque border in the caudal abdomen. There is a slight decrease in the bone density.

31. Draw 0.2 cc of blood for serologic testing for *chlamydia psittaci*.

31. The results will be available in 7 days.

32. Perform a gram stain of the stool.

32. The gram stain reveals an abundance of gram-positive cocci in chains.

33. Perform a fine-needle abdominocentesis.

33. A firm crunch is heard and a thick, yellow proteinaceous fluid is aspirated.

34. Do not perform any diagnostic tests.

34. Go to Section D.

Go to Section D

Section D:

Based on the information you have at this time, what additional procedures would you perform? *(Choose only the procedures you believe relevant to managing the case at this point.)*

35. Anesthetize the bird and perform emergency abdominal surgery.

35. A normal egg is found within an enlarged uterus. The bird dies during surgery. End of problem.

36. Give no treatment and reevaluate in the morning.

36. The bird is found dead in the cage in the morning. End of problem.

37. Administer calcium chloride intravenously.

37. The bird dies during injection. End of problem.

38. Administer an intramuscular dose of doxycycline.

38. There is no improvement.

39. Administer an intramuscular dose of vitamin A and vitamin E .

39. The bird shows slight improvement.

40. Place the bird in a warm incubator.

40. The bird becomes less fluffed.

41. Soak the rump of the bird in a pan of warm water for 10 minutes.	41. The bird fights this procedure.
42. Administer an intramuscular dose of ampicillin and allow the bird to rest.	42. There is no improvement.
43. Give the bird 0.5 cc of a phosphate enema.	43. The bird becomes very ill.
44. Give the bird a subcutaneous dose of warmed lactated Ringer's solution.	44. The bird becomes brighter and more alert.

Go to Section E

Section E:

Based on the results you have obtained so far, what additional treatment might be used to obtain the results you desire? *(Choose only one.)*

45. Squeeze the abdomen to help relieve the feces.	45. Go to Section F.
46. Rub Vaseline on the rump of the bird.	46. Go to Section F.
47. Withhold food from the bird for 12 hours.	47. Go to Section F.
48. Administer an intramuscular dose of calcium gluconate.	48. The bird lays an egg 30 minutes later.
49. Pluck the tail feathers from the bird and wash the vent.	49. Go to Section F.
50. Administer an intramuscular dose of dexamethasone.	50. Go to Section F.
51. Administer an intramuscular dose of diphenhydramine.	51. Go to Section F.

Go to Section F

Section F:

Considering the information you have gained so far, what recommendation would you make to the owner? *(Choose only one.)*

52. Keep the bird on a doxycycline medicated feed for 30 days and return for a recheck exam.	52. End of problem.
53. Supplement the diet with calcium and remove all nesting materials from the cage.	53. End of problem.
54. Continue the seed diet and get a cage mate for the bird.	54. End of problem.
55. Mix diethylstilbestrol into the seed at a dose of 0.10 mg per day for 30 days.	55. End of problem.

56. Change nothing. This is a one-time problem that cannot occur again.

56. End of problem.

57. Euthanize the bird due to the poor prognosis of recovery.

57. End of problem.

END OF PROBLEM

Opening Scene:

A local bird owner calls up and reports that a new bird she purchased about 2 weeks ago is now acting ill. It is a breeder bird and it won't let the owner handle it. She wants to know what she should do.

Go to Section A

Section A:

What directions would you give to the owner regarding bringing the bird in? *(Choose only one.)*

1. Do not bring the bird in. Let it get acclimated for 1 week before coming in.	1. Go to Section B.
2. Place the bird in a paper bag and poke a couple of breathing holes in the bag.	2. Go to Section B.
3. Bring the bird in a clean, sturdy cage.	3. Go to Section B.
4. If possible, bring the bird in its own dirty cage.	4. Go to Section B.
5. Wrap the bird gently in a towel and bring it in.	5. Go to Section B.
6. Place the bird in a thick plastic bag and bring it in.	6. Go to Section B.

Go to Section B

Section B:

The owner has presented the bird. It is a Blue Fronted Amazon. It lays still on the perch with its eyes half open. It does not respond until it is touched. It is unkempt with rough looking feathers and a scaly beak. It is fluffed and shivering, and not very aware of its surroundings. What questions would you like to ask the owner? *(Choose only the questions you believe relevant to managing the case at this point.)*

7. How long have you owned the bird?	7. "For 2 weeks."
8. How many other birds do you have?	8. "I have three breeding pairs of Blue Fronted Amazons that I've owned for 3 years."
9. Are any other birds sick?	9. "No."
10. Where did you get the bird?	10. "From a small pet store downtown."
11. What does the bird eat?	11. "Seeds, fruit, and corn."
12. Have you noticed any change in behavior?	12. "In the past week it has become more depressed, fluffed up, and has not been as active."
13. Has there been a change in appetite?	13. "Yes, it only wants to eat a small amount of corn."

14. Have you noticed any change in the stool?

14. "In the past week, they have become runnier and greener."

15. Have you noticed any change in water intake?

15. "Nope."

16. Do you know whether this bird is captive bred or imported?

16. "No. It didn't come with a leg band."

17. What sex is it?

17. "I don't know. I was going to have it sexed."

18. How old is it?

18. "The shopkeeper said it was 3 years old."

19. Is it on any medications?

19. "No."

20. How long have you been breeding birds?

20. "For 3 years now."

21. Where did you get the cage?

21. "From the bird magazine. It's stainless steel and made for large parrots."

22. How many people live in the house?

22. "Three people."

23. Is anyone in the house ill?

23. "My son has had a cough and fever this past week."

24. Do you have any other pets?

24. "A dog and two cats."

25. Where do you keep the birds?

25. "In the living room next to the kitchen. I put the new bird in a cage with two of the breeder birds to see if they would get along."

Go to Section C

Section C:

Which physical examination procedures would you like to perform at this time? *(Choose only the procedures you believe relevant to managing the case at this point.)*

26. Weigh the bird.

26. The weight is 310 grams (normal 350 to 400 g).

27. Do no physical exam due to the condition of the bird. Place it in a warmed cage and check it in the morning.

27. The bird is worse in the morning.

28. Examine the oral cavity.

28. There is a slight mucoid discharge in the mouth. The choana (respiratory slit) is red and inflamed, and the papillae around the choana are blunted.

29. Palpate the breast muscles and keel.

29. The keel is more prominent than it should be. The bird feels thin.

30. Examine the feathers.

30. The feathers are rough and unkempt, and poorly groomed.

31. Auscultate the heart.

31. The heart rate is 250 beats per minute.

32. Anesthetize the bird with ketamine to finish the exam.

33. Anesthetize the bird with isoflurane to finish the exam.

34. Have the owner hold the bird for the exam.

35. Hold the bird in your bare hands for the exam so you won't hurt it.

36. Palpate the abdomen.

37. Examine the nares.

38. Examine the cage.

39. Examine the stool.

40. Hold the tongue down with your finger to examine the tonsils.

41. Examine the feet.

42. Perform an ophthalmic exam with a direct ophthalmoscope.

43. Palpate the bones of the wing.

44. Auscultate the lungs and air sacs.

45. Palpate the crop.

46. Hold the bird in a large soft towel for the physical exam.

47. Examine the ears.

48. Examine the vent.

49. Obtain rectal temperature.

50. Observe the bird's flight capabilities in the exam room.

32. The bird dies 1 hour later. End of problem.

33. The bird has difficulty under anesthesia, so you stop this procedure.

34. The bird bites the owner on the cheek, and she later sues you for malpractice.

35. The bird inflicts five large bite wounds on your hand.

36. Normal.

37. The nostrils are slightly dilated and have a minor serous discharge.

38. The cage is dirty. There is a full bowl of food.

39. The stool is loose. The feces are soft, and the urates are a bright lime green.

40. The bird bites the tip of your finger off and you have to go to the hospital to have it sewn back on.

41. They appear normal.

42. The pupils are normal. A large oval black mass is noted on the center of the retina in both eyes.

43. Normal.

44. The respiratory rate is 50 and the bird is mildly dyspneic. There is a slight increase in lung sounds bilaterally.

45. The crop is empty.

46. The bird struggles and bites the towel, but the exam continues without problems.

47. They are normal.

48. There is loose stool stuck around the vent.

49. The bird fights this procedure and starts to bleed from the vent.

50. The bird flies into the window and is knocked unconscious. It later recovers.

Go to Section D

Section D:

Based on the information gathered so far, what diagnostic procedures would you like to perform? *(Choose only the procedures you believe relevant to managing the case at this point.)*

51. Do nothing. Advise the owner that the bird will improve in about a week.

51. The owner calls back in 3 days to say the bird is worse.

52. Advise the owner that the bird has ocular melanoma and recommend euthanasia.

52. The owner takes the bird to another vet for a second opinion.

53. Draw 0.2 cc of blood for a complete blood count.

53. The complete blood count results show the following:
    White cell count = 35,000/mm^3
    Heterophil = 25,000/mm^3
    Lymphocytes = 5000/mm^3
    Monocytes = 5000/mm^3
    Some toxic heterophil and bands are noted.
    PCV = 31%
    Total protein = 3.3 g/dl
    There is a marked polychromasia and slight anisocytosis.

54. Draw 0.5 cc of blood for serum chemistries.

54. Serum chemistries are as follows:
    AST = 3500 U/L
    LDH = 850 U/L
    Uric acid = 9.1 mg/dl
    Calcium = 9.0 mg/dl
    Total protein = 3.3 g/dl
    Glucose = 235 mg/dl
    Cholesterol = 199 mg/dl

55. Anesthetize the bird with isoflurane and perform lateral and VD whole body radiographs.

55. The bird has some difficulty with anesthesia, but the x-rays are still taken. There is a bilateral clouding of the air sacs, and a moderate hepatomegaly is present. The lungs have an increased peribronchial density bilaterally.

56. The gram stain reveals >95% gram-positive cocci. The culture results return in 3 days with a light growth of staphylococcus.

56. Perform a gram stain and bacteriological culture of the stool.

57. Submit a bacterial culture from the nares.

57. The culture returns in 3 days with no growth.

58. Submit a fungal culture from the nares.

58. The results will be available in 7 to 10 days.

59. Draw 0.2 cc of blood for Newcastle disease serology.

59. The results will be available in 10 days.

60. Draw 0.5 cc of blood for serology for psittacosis *(Chlamydia psittaci)*.

60. The results return in 5 days with an EBA titer >400 (normal ≤10).

61. Submit 1.5 cc of blood for toxicological analysis.

61. The results will be available in 7 days.

62. Send the bird to the university for a CT scan.

62. The owner refuses this suggestion.

63. Do no more tests. Start bird on calcium EDTA therapy.

63. The bird returns in 3 days considerably worse.

64. Do no more tests. Start bird on oral amoxicillin for 2 weeks.

64. The bird returns in 5 days with no improvement.

65. Anesthetize the bird and submit a cloacal biopsy.

65. The bird has difficulty under anesthesia and bleeds profusely from the biopsy site.

66. Perform a fecal stool flotation.

66. The test is negative.

67. Perform a crop wash and cytology.

67. The cytology is normal.

Go to Section E

Section E:

Based on the results you have obtained so far, what treatment would you recommend for the bird? *(Choose only one.)*

68. Do nothing. Advise the owner no treatment is needed.

68. Go to Section F.

69. Give the bird oral amoxicillin twice daily for 14 days.

69. Go to Section F.

70. Give the bird injectable amoxicillin once daily for 10 days.

70. Go to Section F.

71. Give the bird oral tetracycline daily for 14 days.

71. Go to Section F.

72. Give the bird doxycycline-impregnated food daily for 10 days.

72. Go to Section F.

73. Give the bird doxycycline-impregnated food daily for 45 days.

73. Go to Section F.

74. Give the bird intravenous doxycycline once weekly for 4 weeks.

74. Go to Section F.

75. Give the bird vitamin A injections once weekly for 4 weeks.

75. Go to Section F.

76. Give the bird injectable enrofloxacin twice daily for 10 days.

76. Go to Section F.

77. Give the bird calcium EDTA twice daily for 7 days.

77. Go to Section F.

Go to Section F

Section F:

Based on the information you have acquired, what additional recommendations would you make? *(Choose as many as you feel necessary.)*

78. Advise the owner to sell the bird to avoid further exposure to the other birds.

78. End of problem.

79. Return the bird to the pet store.	79. End of problem.
80. Advise the owner of the zoonotic potential of the disease.	80. End of problem.
81. Euthanize the bird due to the poor prognosis.	81. End of problem.
82. Euthanize all the birds in the household due to the severe contagiousness.	82. End of problem.
83. Test and treat all the birds in the household for the disease.	83. End of problem.
84. Report the disease to the state authorities.	84. End of problem.
85. Sell off all your birds now and start over with new birds.	85. End of problem.
86. Keep the bird in your bird ward in the hospital until it's better.	86. End of problem.
87. Encourage the owner to give the bird to a nursing home since it will never be able to breed.	87. End of problem.
88. Advise the owner that once the bird is treated there is no way it can get the disease again.	88. End of problem.
89. Advise the owner to have her dog tested and treated.	89. End of problem.

END OF PROBLEM

Opening Scene:

A young girl and her father bring in a parakeet to see you. They have had it for a short time and have noticed a change in its appearance. The bird is presented in its cage. It is a small round cage with two bowls of seed and water. There is clean newspaper on the floor of the cage. The girl says that the feet look thorny and the eyes have become crusty.

Go to Section A

Section A:

What questions would you like to ask the girl and her father? *(Choose only the questions you believe relevant to managing the case at this point.)*

1. How old is the bird?

1. "I don't know."

2. How long have you owned it?

2. "Three weeks."

3. When did you first notice the problem?

3. "About 2 weeks ago."

4. What are you feeding it?

4. "Seeds, fruits and veggies, and some sweet potatoes."

5. Where did you get the bird?

5. "At a pet store."

6. How much did the bird cost?

6. "Forty dollars."

7. Has the bird been exposed to any other birds?

7. "It was in with four other parakeets at the pet store."

8. What do the stools look like?

8. "Normal, I guess."

9. Where did you get the cage?

9. "At the pet store."

10. What sex is it?

10. "I don't know."

11. Has there been any change in behavior?

11. "It has become harder to hold it the past week. It seems grouchy."

12. Any change in appetite?

12. "No."

13. Do you have any other pets?

13. "We have a dog. His name is Sparky."

14. Is the bird wild caught or captive bred?

14. "I don't know."

15. Do you have any other birds?

15. "No."

Section B:

Which physical examination procedures would you like to perform at this time? *(Choose only the procedures you believe relevant to managing the case at this point.)*

16. Pluck a feather and examine it under the microscope.

16. The feather appears normal.

17. Weigh the bird.

17. The bird weighs 35 grams (normal).

18. Collect a stool sample for culture.

18. The culture will be available in 4 days.

19. Examine the head and beak.

19. There is proliferation of the tissue of the cere with a honeycomblike appearance to it. There are areas of deep ridges and scales on the beak.

20. Do not examine the bird due to its fragile state.

20. They return in 2 weeks and the problem is worse.

21. Examine the feet.

21. The feet are scaly with small hyperkeratotic thorny projections around the toes.

22. Palpate the breast muscle and keel.

22. Normal.

23. Resect the affected lesion with a small scalpel blade.

23. The bird bleeds profusely from the sight. The girl starts to cry.

24. Soak the affected lesions in mineral oil.

24. The bird returns in 2 days with oil all over its feathers. It is shivering.

25. Examine the feathers.

25. There is a collection of fine white powder down under the contour feathers.

26. Auscultate the lungs and heart.

26. The heart rate is over 300 beats per minute and the respiratory rate is 60 per minute (normal). No abnormalities are heard.

27. Give the bird a week of antibiotics and recheck.

27. They return in 1 week and the bird is worse.

28. Anesthetize the bird with isoflurane to perform a more complete physical exam.

28. The bird has difficulty under anesthesia so you wake it up.

29. Draw 0.10 cc of blood for a psittacosis titer.

29. Results will be available in 7 days.

30. Examine the stool.

30. The feces are firm and regularly shaped. The feces are surrounded by white urates and a small amount of clear urine.

31. Anesthetize the bird with isoflurane and perform an ophthalmic exam.

31. The exam was normal.

32. Give the bird an injection of prednisone and recheck in 1 week.

32. The bird returns in 1 week considerably worse.

33. Examine the mouth and throat with a speculum and tongue depressor.

33. The bird is too small to get the tongue depressor in the mouth.

34. Examine the wings.

34. The skin, bones, and feathers of the wing all appear normal.

Go to Section C

Section C:

Based on the information you have gathered so far, what additional tests or procedures would you like to perform at this time? *(Choose only the procedures you believe relevant to managing the case at this point.)*

35. Draw 0.10 cc of blood for a complete blood count.

35. The complete blood count results are normal.

36. Draw 0.10 cc of blood for psittacosis titer.

36. The lab calls in 1 week and says not enough serum was collected.

37. Draw 0.10 cc of blood for serum chemistries.

37. Only enough blood was obtained to get an AST, which was 85 U/L.

38. Recommend anesthesia and biopsy of the cere.

38. The girl says they can't afford this.

39. Submit a swab of the affected lesions for bacterial culture.

39. The results will be available in 3 days.

40. Recommend anesthesia and biopsy of the feet lesions.

40. The girl says they can't afford this.

41. Perform a squash prep of a newly growing feather.

41. The cytologic exam was normal.

42. Perform a skin scraping of the cere and foot lesion for microscopic exam.

42. The scraping reveals a large amount of keratin and epithelial cells, with numerous large mites. The mites appear to be a *Knemidokoptes* species.

43. Recommend amputation of both feet.

43. The girl starts to cry.

44. Draw 0.10 cc of blood for a serum vitamin A analysis.

44. The lab calls and says they don't do this procedure.

45. No additional tests are needed. Advise the owners the lesions will resolve in about a month.

45. They return and the bird is worse.

46. No additional tests are needed. Send the bird home on a vitamin A supplement.

46. They return and the bird is worse.

47. Perform a corneal scraping with a scalpel blade.

47. The bird wiggles and you cut the eyelid. The girl starts to cry.

48. Examine the powder down of the bird under the microscope.

48. It appears normal under the microscope.

49. Perform a stool gram stain.

49. The gram stain returns normal.

50. Perform an oral gram stain and culture.

50. The results will be available in 4 days.

51. Anesthetize the bird and take skull and foot x-rays.

51. You have difficulty intubating the bird, and the skull is difficult to see with the cone over the bird's head. The feet appear normal.

52. Perform a lead 2 ECG.

52. The ECG registers nothing but interference because the bird is wiggling too much.

53. Submit a fungal culture of the affected lesions.

53. The results will be available in 2 weeks.

Go to Section D

Section D:

With the results you now have, what course of action would you like to take to resolve this problem? *(Choose only one.)*

54. Do nothing. Advise the girl that the problem will go away on its own in about 3 to 4 weeks.

54. End of problem.

55. Advise the girl that the problem will resolve if the bird eats a more well-balanced diet.

55. End of problem.

56. Send the bird home with a daily calcium supplement.

56. End of problem.

57. Send the bird home on a daily vitamin A supplement.

57. End of problem.

58. Send the owner home with a small amount of mineral oil to be applied to the affected lesions daily for 2 weeks.

58. End of problem.

59. Give the bird an IV injection of vitamin A.

59. End of problem.

60. Send the bird home with a daily tetracycline dose to be added to the water for 2 weeks.

60. End of problem.

61. Have the owner spray the bird with a commercial dog and cat flea spray for 2 weeks.

61. End of problem.

62. Administer an oral dose of ivermectin now and repeat it in 2 weeks.

62. End of problem.

63. Send the bird home with a daily dilute chlorhexidine soak and recheck in 2 weeks.

63. End of problem.

64. Have the owners apply clotrimazole to the affected lesions daily for 2 weeks.

64. End of problem.

65. Send the bird home on twice daily injections of enrofloxacin and recheck in 2 weeks.

65. End of problem.

66. Send the bird home on twice daily injections of ivermectin and recheck in 14 days.

66. End of problem.

67. Place the bird in a plastic Ziploc with a small amount of flea powder and shake for about 30 seconds.

67. End of problem.

68. Have the owner place a no pest strip in the cage for 2 weeks.

68. End of problem.

END OF PROBLEM

PROBLEM 4

Opening Scene:

You are a small-animal veterinarian and perform aviary work for a couple of clients. Mrs. Maggie Moody, a well known breeder of English Budgies, calls and says she is having problems with her birds over the past month. She says some birds are looking strange, and she has had a rapid die-off of many young birds. You set up a consultation appointment at her house.

Go to Section A

Section A:

When you arrive, you find that Mrs. Moody has two rooms of parakeets. She put all of the strange-looking and sick birds in one room and the healthy birds are in the basement. What questions would you like to ask Mrs. Moody? *(Choose only the questions you believe relevant to managing the case at this point.)*

1. How many birds do you have?

1. "About 100."

2. How long have you been breeding?

2. "For about 8 years and I have never had a problem."

3. When did the signs start?

3. "About 1 month ago. The new babies had bad feather growth, and some just died about a week after being born."

4. Have you made any recent changes in their environment?

4. "Not that I can think of."

5. Have you changed the cages?

5. "I bought a new cage about 3 months ago."

6. Have you brought any new birds into the collection recently?

6. "I bought four pair of proven breeders from a bird store about 3 months ago."

7. Have you sold any birds recently?

7. "No."

8. Do you have any other bird species in the house?

8. "No."

9. Any change in diet?

9. "No."

10. How many have died?

10. "I lost about 30 in the past month. All but five of them were babies less than 2 weeks old."

11. When did you start separating the birds?

11. "Just this week."

12. How often do you clean the cages?

12. "Once a week."

13. What do you feed them?

13. "A commercial pelleted feed made for budgies."

14. What were the first signs noticed?

14. "The young birds aren't thriving and a lot of them just die. If they don't die, they grow up with poor feather growth and have strange, clubbed, and stunted feathers."

15. Have you had any problems in the past?

15. "None."

Go to Section B

Section B:

Based on the information Mrs. Moody has given you, what procedures would you like to perform next? *(Choose only the procedures you believe relevant to managing the case at this point.)*

16. Observe the healthy birds.

16. There are about 50 birds in an adequately sized, commercial stainless steel cage. They are active and eating. There are five nest boxes in the cage. The room temperature is 75° F. No abnormalities are noticed in their activity or behavior.

17. Observe the ill birds.

17. There are about 20 birds in a large, commercial stainless steel cage. Most of the birds are not flying but are sitting on the floor. Some birds are featherless; the others have deformed feathers. There is one bird on the floor having whole body tremors. The room temperature is 75° F.

18. Weigh each bird with your gram scale.

18. After 4 hours, you record that all the birds weigh between 28 and 40 grams.

19. Examine the owner's breeding records.

19. There is a marked decrease in hatching percentage over the past 2 months. There is also a 400-fold increase in chick mortality over the past 30 days.

20. Examine the cages.

20. They are commercial grade stainless steel aviary cages. They are clean, without rust, and have clean welds with no solder spots.

21. Collect food from both rooms for toxicological analysis.

21. The results will be available in 21 days.

22. Collect water from her tap for lead analysis.

22. The results will be available in 21 days.

23. Perform a test for carbon monoxide in each room.

23. The test is negative. Mrs. Moody complains that you are wasting her time and money.

24. Perform a fungal culture of the cage floor.

24. The culture returns with light growth of a penicillium species.

25. Collect four healthy birds for physical exam.

25. No abnormalities are noted on any of the physical exams. The birds are in good flesh and have normal feathering.

26. Collect four ill birds for physical exam.

26. The birds exhibit decreased feather growth. Several birds have dystrophic feathers on their body. The feathers are twisted and clubbed, or short and lacking good color. One bird has tremors of the head and neck.

27. Collect four dead birds for physical exam.

27. One bird looks completely normal. One chick is underweight with some bruising under the skin. The other two birds have decreased feather growth, abdominal swelling, and subcutaneous hemorrhage.

Go to Section C

Section C:

Based on the information you have gathered so far, what other procedures or diagnostics would you like to perform at this time? (*Choose only the procedures you believe relevant to managing the case at this point.*)

28. Advise the owner to keep the birds separate and sell only the healthy looking birds.

28. She calls in 3 weeks and says 30 more birds have died.

29. Perform a complete blood count and AST on a healthy bird.

29. The complete blood count and AST are normal.

30. Perform a complete blood count and AST on a sick bird.

30. The complete blood count and AST are normal.

31. Perform a stool culture on a sick bird.

31. The culture results return in 3 days with a light growth of staphylococcus.

32. Euthanize all the ill birds and burn the bodies.

32. The owner calls in 3 weeks to report 30 more dead birds.

33. Obtain comparative rectal temperatures of sick and healthy birds.

33. The birds fight this procedure and results are not obtained.

34. Place young sentinel chickens in both rooms for observation for 3 weeks.

34. The chickens are totally normal, and 10 more budgies have died.

35. Submit a dead bird to the state lab for Newcastle disease testing.

35. Results return in 2 weeks as negative.

36. Perform a necropsy and send in tissue samples for histopathology from a dead bird that the owner has kept in her refrigerator for the past 3 days.

36. There is severe autolysis, making the necropsy and histopathology useless.

37. Take two sick birds to your hospital, start them on antibiotics, and place them in your bird ward for further observation.

37. One bird dies 1 week later, and the other bird improves slightly.

38. Freeze two birds, one sick and one healthy, and ship them to the state diagnostic lab for necropsy and histopathology.

38. The state pathologist calls and says results are inconclusive due to autolysis and damage due to freezing of the tissue.

39. Culture the nest boxes for bacteria and fungus.

39. The results return with a positive fungal growth of a penicillium species.

40. Perform a lead analysis of the cages.

40. The results are negative.

41. Euthanize two sick birds and two healthy birds. Necropsy all the birds and submit tissues for histopathology.

41. Both sick birds and one healthy bird have swollen livers with diffuse white dots. They have swollen kidneys, intestinal hemorrhage, cardiomegaly, subcutaneous hemorrhage, and abdominal effusion. The submitted tissues from three of the four birds reveal hepatic necrosis and degeneration, focal renal necrosis, and ballooning degeneration of the skin. Intracellular inclusion bodies are found in all of the tissues from all of the birds submitted.

42. Draw 0.1 cc of blood from five representative birds and submit the combined serum for serology for *Chlamydia psittaci.*

42. The lab calls in 5 days and says the test is invalid due to mixing of the sera.

Go to Section D

Section D:

Based on the information you have acquired so far, what additional test would you like to perform to confirm your suspicions? *(Choose only one.)*

43. Submit swabs of cut tissues of the necropsy specimens, as well as swabs from the cloaca of live birds, for polyomavirus DNA probe analysis.

43. Go to Section E.

44. Submit the livers of euthanized healthy birds to the state diagnostic lab for lead analysis.

44. Go to Section E.

45. Submit the livers of euthanized healthy and ill birds to the state diagnostic lab for lead analysis.

45. Go to Section E.

46. Submit the serum of 10 birds for serological testing for *chlamydia psittaci* (Psittacosis).

46. Go to Section E.

47. Submit the serum of 10 birds for serological testing for avian paramyxovirus (Newcastle disease).

47. Go to Section E.

48. Submit the livers and spleens of healthy and ill birds for herpesvirus isolation and culture at a state approved laboratory.

48. Go to Section E.

Section E:

Based on the information you have acquired so far, what recommendation would you make to the owner? *(Choose only one.)*

49. The disease will run its course. Continue with your breeding operation. The surviving birds will be immune to the disease.

49. End of problem.

50. Place the birds on a doxycycline-impregnated diet for 30 days. Keep the birds in quarantine until done with the treatment.

50. End of problem.

51. Place the birds on calcium EDTA for 7 days, and then recheck the liver lead levels.

51. End of problem.

52. All the birds will eventually die of the disease.

52. End of problem.

53. The healthy birds will remain heathy and should be able to produce healthy offspring next year.

53. End of problem.

54. Sell off all the birds and start over next year with all new birds.

54. End of problem.

55. Depopulate and disinfect the aviary. Restock with well-vaccinated birds or birds that have tested seronegative to this disease.

55. End of problem.

56. Report this disease to the state veterinarian and shut down the breeding operation.

56. End of problem.

57. Thoroughly disinfect both rooms, clean the cages with an antifungal agent, and change the food more frequently.

57. End of problem.

END OF PROBLEM

PROBLEM 5

Opening Scene:

You are a small-animal veterinarian that also sees rabbits and small mammals. A client brings in her 3-year-old castrated male angora rabbit with the complaint that the rabbit has been losing weight. It lays on the table and appears slightly weak, but it responds to handling and it walks well. The owner has 10 rabbits at home and just noticed this rabbit acting sick a couple of days ago.

Go to Section A

Section A:

What questions would you like to ask the owner? *(Choose only the questions you believe relevant to managing the case at this point.)*

1. How long have you owned the rabbit?

2. Any travel history with this rabbit?

3. Are any other rabbits ill?

4. Have you noticed any other problems with this rabbit?

5. Have you noticed any change in the water intake of this rabbit?

6. Is this rabbit with any other rabbits in the same cage?

7. Are you breeding this rabbit?

8. Have you noticed a change in his appetite?

9. How often do you clean the cage?

10. What kind of cage is he in?

11. How often do you change the water?

12. What is the diet?

13. Have you noticed a change in urination?

14. Is he up to date on his vaccinations?

15. Have you noticed any change in the stool?

16. Do you give any vitamin or mineral supplements?

1. "3 Years."

2. "No."

3. "No."

4. "Lately I've noticed he has some hair missing along his sides and on his belly."

5. "No."

6. "Yes, he is with a spayed female."

7. "It's castrated!"

8. "Yes. There has been a gradual decline in his food intake over the past couple of weeks."

9. "Once a week."

10. "It's a commercial stainless steel rabbit cage."

11. "Every other day."

12. "Alfalfa pellets free choice and occasionally a handful of oats."

13. "No."

14. "I didn't think pet rabbits got any vaccinations."

15. "Yes. Lately they have been smaller and there are fewer. They are still round and firm."

16. "No."

| 17. Have you noticed any vomiting? | 17. "No." |
| 18. Have you noticed any coughing or sneezing? | 18. "No." |

Go to Section B

Section B:

Which physical examination procedures would you like to perform at this time? *(Choose only the procedures you believe relevant to managing the case at this point.)*

19. Measure the rectal temperature.	19. The temperature is 39.3°C.
20. Obtain a body weight.	20. The rabbit is underweight at 1.9 kg. (This rabbit should weigh 2.5 kg.)
21. Examine the ears with an otoscope.	21. Normal.
22. Examine the eyes with an ophthalmoscope.	22. Normal.
23. Examine the stool.	23. The stool is small and firm and about half the normal size.
24. Express urine from the bladder.	24. A small amount of urine comes out. It is yellow and cloudy.
25. Examine the skin.	25. There is a moderate alopecia on both sides of the body and on the ventrum of the rabbit. The hairs are broken midshaft and the skin is normal looking.
26. Give 50 mg of ketamine to finish the exam because rabbits can jump and hurt themselves.	26. The rabbit remains asleep for 2 hours.
27. Auscultate the heart and lungs.	27. The heart rate is 190 beats per minute. The respiratory rate is 40. Both sound normal.
28. Auscultate the abdomen.	28. There are decreased gut sounds in all four quadrants of the abdomen.
29. Palpate the abdomen.	29. There is a large doughy mass in the cranial abdomen in the region of the stomach. The caudal abdomen is slightly gassy.
30. Perform a digital rectal exam.	30. The rabbit fights this procedure very much.
31. Palpate the hind legs.	31. They feel normal. The rabbit kicks very hard and scrapes your hand.
32. Hold the rabbit in the air by the front feet to assess hind limb ataxia.	32. The rabbit starts to kick, and it almost breaks its back.

33. Perform an oral exam with a tongue depressor and mouth gag.

33. The rabbit's small mouth won't allow this procedure.

34. Examine the molars of the rabbit by using an otoscope.

34. The molars are even and no sharp points are noted. The gums and cheeks are normal.

Go to Section C

Section C:

Based on the information you have at this time, which diagnostic tests or procedures would you like to perform at this time? (*Choose only the procedures you believe relevant to managing the case at this point.*)

35. Induce vomiting by giving 10 cc of hydrogen peroxide orally.

35. Nothing happens.

36. Induce vomiting by giving 2 cc of syrup of ipecac orally.

36. The rabbit looks uncomfortable but doesn't vomit.

37. Anesthetize the rabbit with ketamine/xylazine to obtain further tests.

37. The rabbit remains asleep for 3 hours.

38. Collect blood for a complete blood count.

38. The complete blood count returns the next day completely normal.

39. Collect serum for a chemistry panel.

39. The BUN is slightly elevated at 33 mg/dl. No other abnormalities are present.

40. Obtain urine for a urinalysis.

40. The urinalysis results are as follows:
The urine specific gravity is 1.035.
pH = 9.0
Negative glucose, ketone, bilirubin, and blood.
The sediment contains a moderate amount of calcium carbonate and struvite crystals.
There are no red or white cells present.

41. Collect a serum sample to screen for laprine gastrointestinal stasis virus (LGSV).

41. Sorry, there is no such thing!

42. Anesthetize the rabbit with isoflurane to obtain the necessary tests.

42. The owner complains that you are doing unnecessary things for such a gentle rabbit that is normally easy to restrain.

43. Do nothing. Advise the owner that the rabbit has a virus infection, which will pass in another week.

43. The rabbit continues to lose weight.

44. Send the rabbit home on a 2 week dose of oral sulfaquinoxaline.

44. The rabbit returns in 1 week with continued weight loss.

45. Obtain lateral and VD abdominal radiographs.

45. The stomach appears enlarged and distended with ingesta. The radiographic appearance of the stomach contents is granular and has a gas pattern surrounding it. There is a small amount of gas in the cecum. There are no other abnormalities.

46. Perform an abdominal ultrasound.

46. There is too much abdominal gas to visualize organs within the abdomen.

47. Perform a skin scraping and fungal culture.

47. The results are negative.

Go to Section D

Section D:

Considering the information you have acquired so far, what treatments are most appropriate? *(Choose only the procedures you believe relevant to managing the case at this point.)*

48. Induce vomiting with 2 cc of syrup of ipecac orally.

48. Nothing happens.

49. Send the rabbit home on a 2 week dose of oral amoxicillin.

49. The rabbit returns in 3 days with a moderate case of diarrhea.

50. Send the rabbit home on a 2 week dose of oral trimethoprim sulfa.

50. The rabbit returns in 1 week with continued weight loss.

51. Anesthetize the rabbit and perform a tooth clipping of the incisors and molars.

51. The rabbit returns in 1 week with continued weight loss.

52. Give an injection of vitamin B to stimulate the appetite.

52. There is no change in the next week.

53. Perform a gentle warm water enema.

53. The rabbit vehemently fights this procedure.

54. Admit the rabbit to your hospital for fluid therapy.

54. Over the next 24 hours, the rabbit is brighter with increased gut sounds.

55. Send the rabbit home on a high phosphorus and low calcium diet to prevent further calciuria.

55. There is no change in the condition.

56. Start the rabbit on a low dose of calcium EDTA until signs dissipate.

56. There is no change in the condition.

Go to Section E

Section E:

What further course of action would you take? *(Choose only one.)*

57. Give the rabbit a lime-sulfur dip for cheyletiella mites.

57. Go to Section F.

58. Advise the owner the problem will correct itself in the next 2 to 3 weeks.

58. Go to Section F.

59. Place all the rabbits on oral lead chelation therapy.

59. Go to Section F.

60. Recommend anesthesia and surgical extraction of trichobezoar if conservative therapy fails.

60. Go to Section F.

61. Recommend euthanasia due to the poor prognosis of gastric neoplasia that commonly occurs in the rabbit.

    61. Go to Section F.

62. Recommend euthanasia due to the poor prognosis of anesthesia and surgery in the rabbit species.

    62. Go to Section F.

63. Euthanize the rabbit due to the possibility of other rabbits contracting this disease.

    63. Go to Section F.

Go to Section F

Section F:

Based on the information you have acquired so far, what recommendation would you make to the owner? *(Choose only one.)*

64. Buy better quality cages from a reputable source to help prevent this problem in all the other rabbits.

    64. End of problem.

65. Destroy all the rabbits because of the contagiousness of this disease.

    65. End of problem.

66. Offer the rabbits a diet higher in fiber and brush them daily.

    66. End of problem.

67. Remove the high calcium diet of alfalfa and replace it with low fiber, high carbohydrate foods such as apples and corn.

    67. End of problem.

68. This problem won't happen again.

    68. End of problem.

69. Perform weekly enemas on the rabbits to prevent further problems.

    69. End of problem.

70. Neuter and spay all the rabbits to prevent the young from contracting this disease.

    70. End of problem.

71. Mixing 2 tablespoons of salt into 4 ounces of water will help prevent this problem from occurring in the other rabbits.

    71. End of problem.

END OF PROBLEM

Opening Scene:

A father and his son bring in a guinea pig (cavy) to be examined. The boy just got the pet about a month ago as a birthday present. They say that over the past week the guinea pig has been reluctant to move and is sneezing a little bit. They brought it in its cage, which is a 10 gallon aquarium. They use cedar chips for bedding, and there is a bowl of guinea pig pellets and water. It is a 4-month-old male cavy. The little boy is very worried about his new pet and is crying when you enter the room.

Go to Section A

Section A:

What questions would you like to ask the owner? (*Choose only the questions you believe relevant to managing the case at this point.*)

1. How long have you owned the guinea pig?

2. Any travel history with this guinea pig?

3. Where did you get him?

4. Have you noticed any other problems with this guinea pig?

5. Have you noticed any change in the water intake of this guinea pig?

6. Do you take the guinea pig out of the cage to play?

7. Do you have any other pets?

8. Have you noticed a change in the appetite?

9. How often do you clean the cage?

10. What is the diet?

11. How often do you change the water?

12. Where do you store the food?

13. Have you noticed a change in urination?

14. Is he up to date on his vaccinations?

15. Have you noticed any change in the stool?

16. Do you give any vitamin or mineral supplements?

1. "For about a month."

2. "No."

3. "At the local pet store."

4. "He's got a runny nose and he isn't eating very well."

5. "No."

6. "About once a day for 15 minutes, but we always watch him closely."

7. "No."

8. "Yes, it's been decreasing the past week."

9. "Once a week."

10. "We bought a bag of guinea pig pellets when we got him."

11. "About once a week."

12. "In the garage."

13. "No."

14. "He doesn't get any shots, does he?"

15. "No."

16. "No."

17. How long have you noticed the signs?

17. "The signs started about 2 weeks ago and they have gotten worse this past week."

18. Have you noticed any coughing or sneezing?

18. "Yes, he's been sneezing a lot."

Go to Section B

Section B:

Which physical examination procedures would you like to perform at this time? *(Choose only the procedures you believe relevant to managing the case at this point.)*

19. Auscultate the heart and lungs.

19. The heart rate is 250 beats per minute and the respiratory rate is 50. The heart and lungs sound normal.

20. Obtain a body weight.

20. The guinea pig weighs 990 grams (normal).

21. Examine the eyes with an ophthalmoscope.

21. Normal.

22. Measure the rectal temperature.

22. The temperature is 38.3°C.

23. Examine the stool.

23. The stool is normal.

24. Examine the nose and nostrils.

24. There is a mild serous nasal discharge.

25. Examine the ears with an otoscope.

25. Normal.

26. Sedate the guinea pig with xylazine to facilitate an easier exam.

26. The guinea pig stays asleep for 2 hours.

27. Observe the cavy walking in the cage.

27. The guinea pig has a very stiff gait and is reluctant to move.

28. Examine the skin.

28. The hair coat is dry, rough, and unkempt.

29. Palpate the abdomen.

29. There is a small amount of gas in the intestines and the guinea pig vocalizes when palpated.

30. Perform a digital rectal exam.

30. The guinea pig starts to cry loudly and the little boy starts to cry again.

31. Palpate the legs.

31. The joints are swollen and the guinea pig cries in pain when the joints are manipulated.

32. Wrap the guinea pig in a towel during the exam to keep it from wiggling.

32. He fights this procedure and examination is difficult.

33. Perform an oral exam with a tongue depressor and mouth gag.

33. The mouth is too small to see anything.

34. Examine the molars of the guinea pig by using an otoscope.

34. The guinea pig struggles a little, but the molars can be visualized. They are even with no points, and the cheek and gums appear normal.

Go to Section C

Section C:

Based on the information you have at this time, which diagnostic tests or procedures would you like to perform? (*Choose only the procedures you believe relevant to managing the case at this point.*)

35. Anesthetize the guinea pig with isoflurane to obtain the necessary tests.

35. This procedure is usually not necessary.

36. Draw blood for serum vitamin E and selenium levels.

36. The lab calls back and says they do not have these tests available.

37. Anesthetize the guinea pig with ketamine/ xylazine to obtain further tests.

37. The guinea pig stays sedated for a very long time.

38. Collect blood for a complete blood count.

38. The complete blood count results are within normal limits.

39. Collect serum for a chemistry panel.

39. The chemistry values are all normal.

40. Obtain urine for a urinalysis.

40. The urinalysis is normal.

41. Draw blood for a serum calcium and phosphorus ratio.

41. The results are within normal limits.

42. Draw blood for a serum vitamin C analysis.

42. The lab calls back and says they do not have these tests available.

43. Do nothing. Advise the owner that this problem will resolve in 1 to 2 weeks.

43. The owners call back in 5 days reporting that the guinea pig is even worse and now has diarrhea.

44. Send the guinea pig home on a 2 week dose of oral ampicillin.

44. The owners call back in 3 days reporting the guinea pig got severe diarrhea and it died. End of problem.

45. Obtain lateral and VD whole body radiographs.

45. The radiographs appear normal except there are enlarged costochondral junctions and the epiphyses of the carpi appear uneven and mildly separated.

46. Perform a culture and sensitivity of the nasal discharge.

46. The results return in 3 days with only normal flora isolated.

47. Sedate the guinea pig and perform a joint tap.

47. The tap reveals normal fluid and some blood present.

Go to Section D

Section D:

Considering the information you have acquired so far, what treatments are most appropriate? *(Choose only the procedures you believe relevant to managing the case at this point.)*

48. Anesthetize the guinea pig and perform a tooth clipping of the incisors and molars.

48. The molars appear normal before the clipping.

49. Start the guinea pig on acyclovir at 10 mg daily for 10 days.

49. There is no change in the cavy's condition.

50. Send the guinea pig home on a 1 week dose of oral trimethoprim sulfa at 15 mg twice daily.

50. The guinea pig returns in 4 days in worse condition.

51. Start the guinea pig on vitamin C at 50 mg daily.

51. The guinea pig rapidly improves over the next 7 days.

52. Give an injection of vitamin B to stimulate the appetite.

52. No improvement is seen.

53. Send the guinea pig home on a 2 week dose of oral amoxicillin.

53. The owners call in 2 days saying the guinea pig has severe diarrhea.

54. Admit the guinea pig to your hospital for fluid therapy.

54. The cavy shows little improvement.

55. Send the guinea pig home on a low phosphorus and high calcium diet.

55. There is no improvement.

56. Start the guinea pig on a low dose of vitamin E and selenium until signs dissipate.

56. There is no improvement.

Go to Section E

Section E:

Based on the information you have acquired so far, what recommendations would you make to the owner? *(Choose only the recommendations you believe to be relevant to the case.)*

57. Recommend euthanasia due to the poor prognosis of ever recovering.

57. The little boy starts to cry.

58. Recommend to the owners to buy fresh guinea pig pellets frequently and to store the food in a cool, dark place.

58. The owners call in 1 month to report that their cavy is doing very well.

59. Daily dietary supplementation of vitamin C will prevent this from recurring.

59. The owners call in 1 month to report that their cavy is doing very well.

60. Recommend anesthesia and tooth clipping if conservative therapy fails.

60. The molars are normal.

61. Daily dietary supplementation of vitamin E and selenium will prevent this from recurring.

62. Recommend euthanasia due to the poor prognosis of anesthesia and surgery in the guinea pig.

63. Euthanize the guinea pig due to the zoonotic potential of the disease.

64. Consider a larger cage that has better ventilation, and change the litter frequently.

65. If given once a week, vitamin C will prevent this problem.

66. Offer the guinea pig a diet higher in fiber.

67. Remove the high calcium diet of pellets and replace it with low fiber, high carbohydrate foods such as oats and corn.

68. Tell the owners that once the guinea pig has been treated, this problem won't happen again.

61. The owners call in 2 weeks to report that the guinea pig died.

62. The little boy starts to cry.

63. The little boy starts to cry.

64. The owners call in 1 month to report that the cavy is doing very well.

65. The owners call in 1 month to report that the cavy is not improving very much.

66. The owners call in 2 weeks to report that the guinea pig is considerably worse and they want to put it to sleep because they think it is suffering.

67. The owners call in 1 week to report that the cavy has severe diarrhea.

68. The owners call back in 2 months to report that the cavy is ill again.

END OF PROBLEM

PROBLEM 7

Opening Scene:

The owner of a 13-year-old spayed domestic shorthair presents the cat to you at your small animal clinic, because he has noticed a progressive weight loss over the previous 2 months. Six months ago the cat weighed 7 kg, but she now weighs approximately 5 kg. The cat's diet consists of dry commercial cat food fed ad libitum. All vaccinations, including rabies and feline leukemia virus, are up to date.

Go to Section A

Section A:

What questions would you ask the owner? *(Choose only the questions you believe relevant to managing the case at this point.)*

1. Have you owned the cat since she was young?	1. "Yes, since she was 3 months old."
2. Does your cat prefer any particular consistency of food (i.e., canned or dry)?	2. "No, she'll eat anything."
3. How has your cat's appetite been?	3. "Her appetite appears to be the same as always, but I can't be sure."
4. Have you noticed any new cats in the neighborhood?	4. "No, there aren't any that I have seen."
5. What type of plants do you have in your home?	5. "All sorts—African violets, spider plants."
6. Has there been any vomiting or diarrhea?	6. "No diarrhea, but she has been vomiting about 3 to 4 times weekly."
7. Have you noticed any sneezing?	7. "Not more than usual."
8. Has there been any change in the water consumption?	8. "I can't be sure since she prefers to drink out of the toilet, but I think she's drinking a lot more."
9. Has there been a change in your cat's activity?	9. "If anything she seems more active than usual."
10. Did anything change in the household 2 months ago?	10. "Nothing has changed in a while."
11. Have you recently started using insecticides or other chemicals on your cat?	11. "No, I don't use that kind of product."
12. Have you noticed any limping recently?	12. "No, she seems to move fine."
13. Is the cat indoor/outdoor or 100% indoor?	13. "She is and always has been 100% indoors."
14. Do you have any other pets?	14. "We have no other pets."
15. Do you ever feed your cat anything besides cat food (e.g., meat)?	15. "No, all she eats is cat food."

• 32 •

16. Does your cat play with toys or small objects?

16. "Yes, she'll occasionally play with small things she finds around."

17. Have you noticed any coughing?

17. "No, not that I've heard."

Go to Section B

Section B:

Which physical examination procedures would you perform at this time? (*Choose only the procedures you believe relevant to managing the case at this point.*)

18. Auscultate the thorax for heart and respiratory sounds.

18. Heart rhythm is regular but with a rate of about 200 beats per minute. Respiratory sounds are normal.

19. Perform a thorough orthopedic examination.

19. No abnormalities are noted.

20. Examine the oral cavity.

20. The oral mucosa is pink, and all the teeth appear normal with mild to moderate gingivitis. No abnormalities are noted.

21. Palpate the neck.

21. Nothing abnormal is noted.

22. Assess postural and spinal reflexes, gait, and proprioception.

22. All reflexes, gait, and proprioception are normal.

23. Palpate the abdomen.

23. You note nothing abnormal.

24. Instill a mydriatic and use an ophthalmoscope to perform a funduscopic examination.

24. The fundus is within normal limits.

25. Use an otoscope to examine the ear canals.

25. The ear canals are normal.

26. Express urine from the bladder.

26. The bladder is empty.

27. Palpate the peripheral lymph nodes.

27. The lymph nodes are of normal size and consistency.

28. Assess the compressibility of the thorax.

28. The thorax compresses normally.

29. Perform a rectal examination.

29. The cat objects greatly, and the rectal cannot be performed.

30. Measure the rectal temperature.

30. The temperature is 38.8°C.

Go to Section C

Section C:

Which diagnostic procedures would you perform? *(Choose only the procedures you believe relevant to managing the case at this point.)*

31. Collect a blood sample for a complete blood count.

32. Collect a serum sample for a serum biochemistry profile.

33. Collect a urine sample for urinalysis.

34. Collect a serum sample for *Toxoplasma* titers.

35. Collect a serum sample for FIP titers.

36. Collect a serum sample for FeLV and FIV titers.

37. Collect a serum sample for measurement of serum amylase concentration.

38. Obtain thoracic radiographs.

39. Obtain abdominal radiographs.

40. Assess cranial nerve function.

31. The complete blood count results show the following:
RBC count = 9 million/mm^3
Hemoglobin = 13 gm/dl
PCV = 41%
Platelets = 350,000/mm^3
Total WBC = 9800/mm^3
Neutrophils = 7900/mm^3
Lymphocytes = 1400/mm^3
Monocytes = 400/ mm^3
Eosinophils = 100/ mm^3

32. The blood chemistry profile shows:
Glucose = 180 mg/dl
BUN = 20 mg/dl
Creatinine = 1.6 mg/dl
Calcium = 9.0 mg/dl
Phosphorus = 5.1 mg/dl
Total protein = 6.4 g/dl
Albumin = 3.0 g/dl
Globulin = 3.4 g/dl
Sodium = 153 mEq/L
Potassium = 4.5 mEq/L
Chloride = 120 mEq/L
t. bilirubin = 0.1 mg/dl
ALT = 220 IU/L
ALP = 300 IU/L
AST = 40 IU/L

33. Unfortunately, a urine sample cannot be obtained, because the bladder is empty.

34. The IgG and IgM titers are both negative.

35. The FIP titer is negative.

36. The FIV and FeLV are negative.

37. The amylase is 1500 IU/L.

38. The thorax is within normal limits.

39. There is air in the stomach; otherwise, the abdomen is within normal limits.

40. The assessment of all cranial nerves is normal.

41. Perform an electrocardiogram.

41. The rhythm is a sinus tachycardia.

42. Obtain a stool sample for examination for parasites.

42. The fecal is negative.

43. Obtain a stool sample for fecal cytology.

43. There is a mixed population of bacteria; no cells are seen.

44. Obtain a serum sample for trypsinlike immunoreactivity assay.

44. The trypsinlike immunoreactivity is 30 μg/L.

45. Obtain a serum sample for thyroxine (T_4) assay.

45. The T_4 is 3.9 μg/dl.

Go to Section D

Section D:

Considering the information you have gained so far, which further diagnostic procedures would you perform? *(Choose only the procedures you believe relevant to managing the case at this point.)*

46. Administer 1 unit of ultralente insulin and perform a 24 hour glucose curve.

46. The cat's blood glucose drops to 50 mg/dl after 12 hours.

47. Obtain pre- and postprandial serum samples for determination of bile acid concentrations.

47. The pre- and postprandial bile acids are 5 and 10 μM/L, respectively.

48. Perform an ultrasound of the liver.

48. There are some very mild changes in the echogenicity of the liver, most likely changes associated with old age.

49. Obtain an ultrasound-guided biopsy of the liver.

49. The biopsies are within normal limits.

50. Perform an abdominal exploratory to obtain gastric, intestinal, and liver biopsies.

50. At exploratory, the abdominal contents appear normal, and all biopsies obtained are within normal limits.

51. Perform endoscopy to obtain biopsies of the stomach and proximal small intestine.

51. At endoscopy, there is a lot of hair in the stomach. The biopsies of the stomach and duodenum are within normal limits.

52. Obtain a serum sample for determination of the concentration of steroid-induced isoenzyme of alkaline phosphatase.

52. Cats do not have a steroid-induced isoenzyme.

53. Obtain a sample of feces for culture.

53. The culture contains a mix of gram-positive and gram-negative bacteria.

54. Perform an upper GI contrast study.

54. The transit time of the barium through the stomach and small intestine is normal. No abnormalities are noted with the exception of the presence of a hair ball in the stomach.

55. Perform a T_3 suppression test.

55. The T_4 before T_3 administration is 3.9 μg/dl; after T_3 the T_4 is 3.7 μg/dl. The T_3 was measured before and after administration to ensure that the T_3 had been administered and the serum concentrations increased appropriately.

Go to Section E

Section E:

What course of action would you take? *(Choose only one.)*

56. Send the cat home on 0.5 U ultralente insulin daily and tell the owner to return in 1 week for another glucose curve.

56. End of problem.

57. Tell the owner the cat's problems are probably age-related, but she should bring the cat back in 4 weeks if the cat gets worse.

57. End of problem.

58. Tell the owner no definitive diagnosis can be found. The cat's problems are probably age-related and nothing to worry about.

58. End of problem.

59. Prescribe methimazole for the cat at 5 mg twice daily per os and tell the owner the cat should be seen in 2 weeks for a recheck.

59. End of problem.

60. Prescribe a laxative to take care of the hair balls and tell the owner to feed the cat a bland diet.

60. End of problem.

61. Tell the owner you are concerned about the gingivitis. Since the cat is in relatively good health, you recommend a dental examination be performed and then assess if this helps with the problem.

61. End of problem.

END OF PROBLEM

Opening Scene:

The owner of a 4-year-old spayed Labrador retriever presents the dog to you at your small animal clinic for a second opinion. The dog has a waxing and waning history over the past 3 months. The first thing the owner notices is that the dog's appetite slowly decreases over 2 to 3 days, then she starts vomiting. Each time this occurs, the dog has been taken to her usual veterinarian. She is usually hospitalized and within 1 to 2 days is better. However, within 1 to 2 weeks the signs recur. This has happened about four to five times in the past, and she has not been eating for the past day. There are no other pets in the household.

GO TO SECTION A

Section A:

What questions would you ask the owner? (*Choose only the questions you believe relevant to managing the case at this point.*)

1. When was the last time the dog was vaccinated?

   1. "She was vaccinated about 7 months ago."

2. When outside is the dog allowed to roam, is she in a fenced yard, or is she on a leash?

   2. "She never goes outside unsupervised. She is always in our fenced yard or being walked on a leash."

3. What type of treatment was given to your dog while she was hospitalized by the other veterinarian?

   3. "It seems as if there was a different treatment every time—different antibiotics, prednisone, antivomiting medicine. She was also getting some type of fluid by injection."

4. Is she on any medication currently?

   4. "No, she was never sent home with any medication because she always seemed better when she was discharged."

5. Has she been tested for heartworm or is she on preventative?

   5. "She was last tested for heartworm about 2 years ago, and then was on preventative for that season. We meant to get her tested again at the beginning of this season, but then all this started."

6. What is her usual diet?

   6. "She usually gets fed two meals daily of quality dry dog chow."

7. Have you noticed any diarrhea?

   7. "During a couple of episodes, she has had soft stools."

8. Has there been any change in her water consumption?

   8. "She seems to be drinking a little more than usual."

9. Have you noticed any limping or difficulty walking?

   9. "No, I haven't noticed any limping, but during her episodes she does seem to be reluctant to climb stairs."

10. Has there been any nasal discharge?

    10. "No, there has not been any nasal discharge."

11. Did anything unusual happen in your household before the first episode occurred?

    11. "Not that I can think of."

12. Does she often get fed table scraps?

12. "We try not to give her table food, but every once in a while a guest will indulge her or we'll give her a special treat. It's pretty uncommon."

13. How long have you owned her?

13. "We've owned her ever since she was a puppy."

14. What is her usual activity level and has that changed?

14. "She is usually a very active dog, but she seems less active ever since these episodes started."

15. Has her weight changed over the past 3 months?

15. "I think she looks thinner than she used to."

16. Has there been any coughing?

16. "No, I don't think I've heard any coughing."

17. Has she escaped from the yard or house lately?

17. "No, there haven't been any escapes."

18. Has there been any change in her urination habits?

18. "Well, I guess she does ask to go out more than she used to, but usually we just let her out in the yard and don't watch to see what she is doing."

19. Has there ever been any difficulty in passing stool (e.g., straining)?

19. "No, she has never had a problem while we were watching her, even when the stool was soft."

20. Have you been using any flea products or other insecticides/parasiticides lately?

20. "Yes, we've sprayed her once or twice a month with some type of flea spray, and she usually wears a flea collar."

Go to Section B

Section B:

Which physical examination procedures would you perform at this time? (*Choose only the procedures you believe relevant to managing the case at this point.*)

21. Measure the rectal temperature.

21. The rectal temperature is 37.9°C.

22. Dilate the pupils and perform a funduscopic examination.

22. The fundus is within normal limits.

23. Auscultate the thorax for heart and respiratory sounds.

23. The respiratory sounds are within normal. The heart rate is 50 beats per minute, and the rhythm is regular. There are no murmurs.

24. Palpate the trachea, trying to elicit a cough.

24. The trachea palpates normally, and no cough can be elicited easily.

25. Perform a rectal examination.

25. The rectal examination is normal.

26. Palpate the abdomen.

26. Abdominal palpation is normal. A few bowel loops feel mildly dilated.

27. Examine the oral cavity.

27. The teeth and gums are nonremarkable. The mucous membranes appear slightly pale.

28. Assess the peripheral lymph nodes.

28. The lymph nodes are all normal.

29. Perform a complete orthopedic examination.

29. No abnormalities are found in the forelimbs. When palpating the rear limbs, the dog seems more tense. No pain is shown, but it is difficult to obtain a full range of movement in the joints due to the lack of cooperation.

30. Assess postural and spinal reflexes and proprioception.

30. The reflexes and proprioception are normal.

31. Carefully palpate all thoracolumbar vertebra for signs of pain and asymmetry.

31. There is no sign of pain, and all vertebrae appear symmetrical.

32. Assess the cranial nerves.

32. All cranial nerves appear normal.

33. Palpate each rear limb to assess the femoral pulses.

33. The femoral pulses are strong, symmetrical, and synchronous with the heartbeat.

34. Perform a digital vaginal examination.

34. No abnormalities are noted.

Go to Section C

Section C:

Which diagnostic procedures would you perform? (*Choose only the procedures you believe relevant to managing the case at this point.*)

35. Sedate the dog and carefully palpate the rear limbs for abnormalities.

35. No abnormalities are noted.

36. Collect a serum sample for a complete biochemical profile.

36. The blood chemistry profile shows:
Glucose = 80 mg/dl
BUN = 85 mg/dl
Creatinine = 2.8 mg/dl
Calcium = 9.0 mg/dl
Phosphorus = 6.8 mg/dl
Total protein = 7.8 g/dl
Albumin = 4.4 g/dl
Globulin = 3.4 g/dl
Sodium = 137 mEq/L
Potassium = 6.7 mEq/L
Chloride = 95 mEq/L
t. bilirubin = 0.1 mg/dl
ALT = 80 IU/L
ALP = 120 IU/L
AST = 25 IU/L

37. Collect a blood sample for a complete blood count.

37. The complete blood count results show the following:
RBC count = 4.8 million/mm^3
Hemoglobin = 11 g/dl
MCV = 62 fl
MCHC = 34 g/dl
PCV = 32%
Platelets = 205,000/mm^3
Total WBC = 12,400/mm^3

Neutrophils = 8100/mm^3
Lymphocytes = 2300/mm^3
Monocytes = 1200/mm^3
Eosinophils = 800/mm^3

38. Collect a urine sample for urinalysis.

38. It is a free-catch urine sample.
Specific gravity = 1.012
pH = 7.5
Glucose = negative
Ketones = negative
Protein = 1+
Blood = negative
RBC = 0-1/hpf
WBC = 2-3/hpf
Bacteria = occasional
Casts = 0-1 hyaline cast/hpf
Crystals = 1+ struvite

39. Collect a serum sample for thyroxine (T$_4$) and triiodothyronine (T$_3$) assay.

39. The T$_4$ is 1.1 µg/dl and the T$_3$ is 20 ng/dl.

40. Collect a serum sample for determination of serum amylase and lipase concentrations.

40. The serum amylase is 890 IU/L and the lipase is 215 IU/L.

41. Obtain radiographs of the pelvis.

41. The pelvis is within normal limits.

42. Obtain radiographs of the abdomen.

42. There are a few mildly dilated loops of bowel. Otherwise, the abdomen appears within normal limits.

43. Perform a Knott's test and occult heartworm test.

43. Both heartworm tests are negative.

44. Obtain a stool sample for fecal cytology.

44. There is a mixed population of bacteria, and there are no abnormal cells.

45. Obtain a stool sample for fecal flotation.

45. No parasites or parasite ova are seen.

46. Perform an ultrasonographic examination of the abdomen.

46. There are a few mildly dilated loops of bowel. Otherwise, the abdomen appears within normal limits.

47. Collect a blood sample for lead assay.

47. The lead level is nondetectable.

48. Perform gastric lavage to try to obtain samples of stomach contents for toxicant analysis.

48. No stomach contents are obtained.

49. Obtain an electrocardiogram (ECG).

49. The heart rate is 50. It is a sinus rhythm; however, the T waves are tall and peaked.

50. Obtain a urine sample by cystocentesis and submit it for bacterial culture.

50. The urine culture is negative.

51. Obtain radiographs of the thorax.

51. The heart appears smaller than normal. All else is within normal limits.

Go to Section D

Section D:

Considering the information you have gained so far, which further diagnostic procedures would you perform? *(Choose only the procedures you believe relevant to managing the case at this point.)*

52. Collect a blood level to determine cholinesterase activity.

52. Cholinesterase activity is within normal limits.

53. Perform a low dose dexamethasone suppression.

53. The baseline cortisol is 1.1 µg/dl. At 4 and 8 hours postdexamethasone, the cortisol is <1 µg/dl.

54. Perform a thyroid-stimulating hormone (TSH) response test.

54. The baseline T_4 is 1.2 µg/dl, and the post-TSH level is 4.5 µg/dl.

55. Perform an upper gastrointestinal contrast study.

55. No abnormalities are noted.

56. Perform an endoscopy to obtain biopsies of the stomach and proximal small intestine.

56. No gross abnormalities are noted. The biopsies are within normal limits.

57. Obtain a blood sample for reticulocyte count.

57. The reticulocyte count is 55,000/mm³.

58. Perform an ACTH stimulation (ACTH response test).

58. The pre-ACTH cortisol is 1.1 µg/dl and the post-ACTH cortisol is 1.2 µg/dl.

59. Perform a bone marrow aspirate and submit the sample for cytology.

59. All blood line precursors appear in normal numbers and morphology. There is no sign of red blood cell regeneration.

60. Obtain an echocardiographic study.

60. The heart is normal.

61. Perform an intravenous pyelogram (excretory urogram).

61. The kidneys appear normal.

Go to Section E

Section E:

What course of action would you take? *(Choose only one.)*

62. Inform the owners that the dog has renal failure of unknown cause. Recommend a protein-restricted diet and phosphate binders and tell the owners you need to recheck the dog in 2 weeks.

62. End of problem.

63. Inform the owners that the dog has a mild anemia. Prescribe iron supplements and anabolic steroids and recommend a recheck in 4 weeks.

63. End of problem.

64. Inform the owners that the dog has Addison's disease. Prescribe fludrocortisone acetate and tell the owners that the dog needs to be rechecked in 5 days.

64. End of problem.

65. Inform the owners that the dog appears to have a sensitive stomach since no cause for the anorexia and vomiting can be found. Recommend a hypo-allergenic, bland diet and tell the owners you want to recheck the dog in 4 weeks.

65. End of problem.

66. Inform the owners that the dog appears to have a sensitive stomach since no cause for the anorexia and vomiting can be found. Prescribe metoclo-pramide for the owners to give at home the next time an episode occurs, and ask them to call you to let you know if it helps.

66. End of problem.

END OF PROBLEM

Opening Scene:

A 10-year-old castrated male domestic shorthair is brought to you at your small animal hospital, because the owner thinks that the cat is spending a lot of time in the litter box. The cat seems to go in there to urinate much more often than he used to. Over the last couple of days, the cat seems depressed and his appetite has decreased. The cat has belonged to the same owner his whole life. He is a 100% indoor cat, and there are no other pets in the household.

Go to Section A

Section A:

What questions would you ask the owner? *(Choose only the questions you believe relevant to managing the case at this point.)*

1. When was the last time your cat was vaccinated?

   1. "He was vaccinated 7 months ago."

2. What is his usual diet?

   2. "He is fed a lowfat, high fiber diet because he tends to be overweight."

3. Have you noticed any change in his stools?

   3. "Not really, but I don't pay that much attention to the stool when I clean the litter box. They're certainly formed."

4. Has there been any change in urine volume?

   4. "It seems that there is an increase in the volume."

5. Do you think he is usually urinating or defecating when he is in the litter box?

   5. "I think he's urinating."

6. Has there been any change in his appetite previous to the last couple of days?

   6. "He was eating a little bit less than he used to, but he's also less active."

7. Does he ever seem uncomfortable when he is in the litter box?

   7. "No, there's no crying or anything. He's just in there a long time."

8. Have you noticed any vomiting?

   8. "For a couple of days before he started acting depressed, I noticed that he vomited about 4 to 6 times, but that seems to have stopped now. He typically vomits 2 to 3 times a month."

9. Has there been any change in his weight?

   9. "No change that I've noticed."

10. Has there been a diet change recently?

    10. "No, he's always eaten the R/d dry."

11. Has there been any recent exposure to other cats?

    11. "I don't think so. He hasn't been boarded or anything and he doesn't go outside."

12. Do you ever feed raw meat to your cat?

    12. "No, he gets no table scraps."

13. Have there ever been any episodes in the past where the cat seemed to be using the litter box frequently?

    13. "No, I've never noticed him do this before."

14. Does your cat play with small objects or toys?	14. "He plays with all sorts of things—whatever he can find, unfortunately."
15. Is your cat still able to jump normally and hold his tail erect?	15. "I think so."
16. Is there any possibility of trauma (e.g., someone hitting the cat or the cat getting slammed in a door)?	16. "Not that I know of."
17. Has there been any change in his activity?	17. "I think he's a little bit less active recently, but I attributed that to age."

Go to Section B

Section B:

Which physical examination procedures would you perform at this time? *(Choose only the procedures you believe relevant to managing the case at this point.)*

18. Measure the rectal temperature.	18. The temperature is 38.4°C.
19. Perform a thorough neurological examination.	19. The cat is extremely uncooperative, but there are no major abnormalities noted.
20. Express urine from the bladder.	20. The cat objects at first, but you are able to express a small amount of urine. It looks grossly normal.
21. Palpate the abdomen.	21. The kidneys feel small and their surface is irregular. The bladder is midsize, soft, and nonpainful.
22. Palpate the neck.	22. There are no abnormalities noted.
23. Auscultate the thorax for heart and respiratory sounds.	23. The lungs sound clear. The heart rate is 140 beats per minute and regular.
24. Carefully palpate the tail for any sign of vertebral trauma and assess pain perception.	24. The tail is being held erect throughout the history-taking period. No abnormalities are noted on examination.
25. Assess the compressibility of the thorax.	25. The thorax compresses as expected.
26. Palpate all peripheral lymph nodes.	26. All lymph nodes are within normal limits.
27. Examine the oral cavity.	27. The mucous membranes are pink. There is mild gingivitis.
28. Determine hydration status by assessing skin turgor over the dorsal and lateral thorax.	28. The skin turgor is decreased, and you estimate the cat to be 5% to 7% dehydrated.

29. Perform a rectal examination.

29. The cat objects greatly. A small amount of blood is noted on your finger when you're done, but no abnormalities were noted during the rectal.

30. Express the anal sacs.

30. The contents of the anal sacs appear normal.

Go to Section C

Section C:

Which diagnostic procedures would you perform? *(Choose only the procedures you believe relevant to managing the case at this point.)*

31. Collect a serum sample for a complete biochemical profile.

31. The blood chemistry profile shows the following:
Glucose = 135 mg/dl
BUN = 150 mg/dl
Creatinine = 4.0 mg/dl
Calcium = 9.0 mg/dl
Phosphorus = 8.0 mg/dl
Total protein = 8.0 g/dl
Albumin = 4.6 g/dl
Globulin = 3.4 g/dl
Sodium = 150 mEq/L
Potassium = 4.4 mEq/L
Chloride = 106 mEq/L
t. bilirubin = 0.1 mg/dl
ALT = 25 IU/L
ALP = 36 IU/L
AST = 25 IU/L
tCO_2 = 14 mEq/L

32. Collect a blood sample for a complete blood count.

32. The complete blood count results show the following:
RBC count = 4.1 million/mm^3
Hemoglobin = 10 g/dl
MCV = 43 fl
MCHC = 36 g/dl
PCV = 29%
Platelets = 205,000/mm^3
Total WBC = 8700/mm^3
Neutrophils = 5100/mm^3
Lymphocytes = 3300/mm^3
Monocytes = 200/mm^3
Eosinophils = 100/mm^3

33. Collect a urine sample for urinalysis.

33. It is a cystocentesis urine sample.
Specific gravity = 1.012
pH = 7.5
Glucose = negative
Ketones = negative
Protein = negative
Blood = negative
RBC = 0-1/hpf
WBC = 2-3/hpf
Bacteria = none

Casts = 0-1 hyaline cast/hpf
Crystals = 2+ struvite

34. Obtain radiographs of the thorax.

35. Collect a serum sample for thyroxine (T₄) and triiodothyronine (T₃) assay.

36. Submit a urine sample for determination of urinary protein:creatinine ratio.

37. Obtain radiographs of the abdomen.

38. Sedate the cat to perform an in-depth ophthalmoscopic exam and to measure a direct femoral blood pressure.

39. Perform a thyrotropin-releasing hormone (TRH) response test.

40. Obtain an ultrasonographic examination of the abdomen.

41. Perform a double contrast radiographic study of the bladder.

42. Perform a water deprivation test.

43. Collect a urine sample to be submitted for bacterial culture.

44. Collect a serum sample for determination of FeLV and FIV status.

45. Collect a serum sample for determination of FIP titer.

46. Obtain a bone marrow aspirate and submit the sample for cytology.

47. Obtain a blood sample for assessment of coagulation.

48. Obtain a blood sample from the femoral artery for assessment of blood gases.

34. No abnormalities are noted.

35. The T_4 is 2.0 μg/dl and the T_3 is 25 ng/dl.

36. The protein:creatinine ratio is 0.6.

37. The abdominal contents are within normal limits with the exception of the kidneys. Both appear small and irregular. Formed stool is noted within the colon that is more radiodense than average, suggesting that it is drier than normal.

38. The only abnormality noted is enlarged, tortuous retinal vessels and a small petechial hemorrhage in the left eye. The direct blood pressure reading is inaccurate due to the sedation.

39. The results of the test are within normal limits.

40. The kidneys are small and pitted. The medullary/cortical junction is indistinct, and the medulla has an increased echogenicity. There are crystals noted in the urinary bladder.

41. The bladder and urethra are normal.

42. The cat rapidly dehydrates, becomes very depressed, and vomits repeatedly.

43. The culture is negative for aerobic bacteria.

44. The ELISA for FeLV and FIV are negative.

45. The titer for FIP is 1:200.

46. All cell lines are present within the bone marrow. The red cells are not showing signs of regeneration (e.g., hyperplasia), but the maturation sequence is normal.

47. All coagulation parameters are within normal limits.

48. The blood gas results show the following:
pH = 7.28
PaO_2 = 90 mm Hg

$$PCO_2 = 40 \text{ mm Hg}$$
$$HCO_3 = 13 \text{ mEq/L}$$

49. Obtain a blood sample and submit for determination of reticulocyte count.

49. There are fewer than 60,000 reticulocytes/μl.

50. Instill a mydriatic and use an ophthalmoscope to perform a funduscopic examination.

50. The retinal vessels are slightly enlarged and tortuous. A petechial hemorrhage is noted in the left eye.

51. Determine the systolic blood pressure using a Doppler sphygmomanometer.

51. Using the Doppler sphygmomanometer, the systolic pressure is measured to be 200 mm Hg.

Go to Section D

Section D:

Considering the information you have gained so far, which treatments are most appropriate? *(Choose any treatments you believe relevant to resolving the animal's problem.)*

52. Administer a soap and warm water enema to the cat.

52. The cat passes some firm stool shortly after the enema.

53. Administer furosemide at 0.5 mg/kg IV every 8 to 12 hours.

53. The cat continues to urinate a large amount of urine.

54. Administer erythropoietin SQ and inform the owner this will need to be continued for the life of the cat.

54. The PCV increases slightly over a few weeks time. No difference is noted in the cat's attitude.

55. Calculate the bicarbonate dose required to correct the acidosis and administer to the cat IV over 6 to 8 hours.

55. The pH returns to normal.

56. Administer an IM injection of ferrous sulfate and stanazolol and dispense iron and stanazolol tablets to be given at home.

56. No improvement is noted.

57. Dispense amoxicillin/clavulanic acid (13.75 mg/kg) to be given at home twice daily for 10 days.

57. The cat continues to urinate large amounts of urine. No improvement is noted.

58. Place a urinary catheter to make sure the cat is urinating.

58. Urine passes freely through the catheter.

59. Place an IV catheter and administer fluids at two to four times maintenance.

59. Over 2 days, the BUN and creatinine decrease to 80 mg/dl and 2.9 mg/dl, respectively. The cat is feeling much better. The fluids are slowly discontinued, and the cat is discharged.

60. Perform a crossmatch and administer a blood transfusion.

60. No change is noticed in the cat's attitude.

61. Administer an antidiuretic hormone and monitor the urine specific gravity to determine if the cat can concentrate its urine.

61. The urine does not become concentrated.

62. Dispense prednisone to be given at 0.5 mg/kg every 12 hours for 10 days.

62. No change is noted in the cat's urination habits or attitude.

63. Dispense amlodipine to be given at 0.625 mg daily.

63. After 2 weeks therapy, the cat's systolic blood pressure is 120 mm Hg.

Go to Section E

Section E:

Which course of action would you take? *(Choose all that are appropriate.)*

64. Recommend euthanasia since the cat has renal failure.

64. End of problem.

65. Recommend limiting the cat's access to water so that it will not drink too much.

65. End of problem.

66. Recommend a diet change to a protein-restricted diet.

66. End of problem.

67. Recommend a diet change to a diet designed to treat cats that have urinary crystals.

67. End of problem.

68. Inform the owner that the cat has FIP. Inform the owner you want to recheck the cat periodically, and prednisone therapy may need to be lifelong.

68. End of problem.

69. Recommend euthanasia since the cat has FIP.

69. End of problem.

70. Inform the owner you want to recheck the cat in 10 days in order to determine if the cat still has many crystals in its urine.

70. End of problem.

71. Inform the owner you want to recheck the cat in 10 days to obtain a blood sample for a complete blood count and a reticulocyte count.

71. End of problem.

72. Inform the owner you want to recheck the cat in 10 days to reevaluate BUN and creatinine.

72. End of problem.

END OF PROBLEM

Opening Scene:

A 9-year-old intact male Springer spaniel is brought to you because the owners have noticed swelling in all four feet. They moved to your town in New York about 6 weeks ago at the beginning of December. The swelling has been present for about 1 week. They gave the dog some aspirin at home, thinking the cold was causing a joint problem, and that may have helped a little. The dog is current on vaccinations (rabies and distemper/parvo/parainfluenza/leptospira/adenovirus).

Go to Section A

Section A:

What questions would you ask the owner? *(Choose only the questions you believe relevant to managing the case at this point.)*

1. Does your dog ever limp?

2. How has your dog's activity been?

3. Has there been any change in his appetite?

4. Have you noticed any nasal discharge?

5. Has there been any coughing?

6. When was your dog checked for heartworm?

7. Has there been any change in his weight recently?

8. Have you ever traveled with your dog?

9. From where did you move?

10. Are any of your new neighbors unhappy that you have a dog?

11. Has there been any vomiting or diarrhea?

12. Is your dog currently on any medications?

13. Do you think your dog ever has difficulty hearing?

14. Has your dog ever had a problem like this in the past?

---

1. "No, we've never seen him limp."

2. "His activity seems to have been decreasing over a period of months. We noticed a decrease even before we moved."

3. "His appetite isn't as good as it used to be."

4. "Not that we've seen."

5. "Now that you mention it, he has been coughing lately."

6. "He was checked about 2 years ago, I think, and put on the daily preventive."

7. "He looks a little thinner, maybe."

8. "We've taken him to the Jersey shore a few times over the years."

9. "We moved from another town in New York about 30 miles from here."

10. "Not that we're aware of."

11. "Not to our knowledge."

12. "The only thing he has received recently is the aspirin."

13. "No, he seems to hear clearly."

14. "No, he really has been a very healthy dog up until now."

15. Has your dog ever been bred?

15. "Yes, he's under contract to the breeder who sold him to us. She uses him for breeding about once a year. He was bred about 8 months ago."

16. Do you have any other pets?

16. "No, he's the only one."

17. Has there been any change in water consumption?

17. "He has never been a big drinker, and I don't think that has changed."

Go to Section B

Section B:

Which physical examination procedures would you perform at this time? *(Choose only the procedures you believe relevant to managing the case at this point.)*

18. Perform a thorough orthopedic examination.

18. The distal joints (carpi and tarsi) are difficult to palpate due to the swelling. All other joints appear normal.

19. Palpate all peripheral lymph nodes.

19. All lymph nodes are within normal limits.

20. Perform an ophthalmological exam, including visualization of the fundus.

20. The examination is normal.

21. Examine the oral cavity.

21. The mucous membranes are pink. No abnormalities are seen.

22. Assess the femoral pulses.

22. The femoral pulses are synchronous with the heartbeat, strong and symmetrical.

23. Perform a rectal examination.

23. The prostate is mildly to moderately enlarged. It is nonpainful and symmetrical, and the median raphe can be distinguished.

24. Palpate the abdomen.

24. No abnormalities are noted.

25. Attempt to inspect the nasal cavity with an otoscope.

25. The dog objects greatly, and in the struggle develops epistaxis.

26. Inspect the ear canals and tympanic membranes.

26. The ear canals and tympanic membranes are normal.

27. Auscultate the thorax for heart and respiratory sounds.

27. The lung sounds are clear. The heart rate is 120 beats per minute and regular.

28. Examine the distal extremities at the site of the swelling.

28. The swelling is cool and nonpainful. The areas of swelling pit easily, but the pits resolve quickly. The swelling involves the feet and extends to the distal radius in the front and the distal tibia in the rear.

29. Assess postural and spinal reflexes, gait, and proprioception.

29. All are within normal limits.

30. Measure the rectal temperature.

30. The temperature is 37.7°C.

Go to Section C

Section C:

Which diagnostic procedures would you perform? *(Choose only the procedures you believe relevant to managing the case at this point.)*

31. Collect a serum sample for a complete biochemical profile.

31. The blood chemistry profile shows:
   Glucose = 92 mg/dl
   BUN = 18 mg/dl
   Creatinine = 1.1 mg/dl
   Calcium = 7.0 mg/dl
   Phosphorus = 3.7 mg/dl
   Total protein = 7.0 g/dl
   Albumin = 1.1 g/dl
   Globulin = 5.9 g/dl
   Sodium = 149 mEq/L
   Potassium = 5.1 mEq/L
   Chloride = 118 mEq/L
   t. bilirubin = 0.3 mg/dl
   ALT = 25 IU/L
   ALP = 320 IU/L
   AST = 25 IU/L
   tCO_2 = 22 mEq/L

32. Collect a blood sample for a complete blood count.

32. The complete blood count results show the following:
   RBC count = 8.2 million/mm^3
   Hemoglobin = 15 g/dl
   MCV = 67 fl
   MCHC = 36 g/dl
   PCV = 45%
   Platelets = 355,000/mm^3
   Total WBC = 17,200/mm^3
   Neutrophils = 12,800/mm^3
   Lymphocytes = 1700/mm^3
   Monocytes = 900/mm^3
   Eosinophils = 1800/mm^3

33. Collect a urine sample for urinalysis.

33. It is a free-catch urine sample.
   Specific gravity = 1.023
   pH = 6.5
   Glucose = negative
   Ketones = negative
   Protein = 3+
   Blood = negative
   RBC = 0-1/hpf
   WBC = 2-3/hpf
   Bacteria = occasional
   Casts = none
   Crystals = occasional calcium oxalate

34. Collect a serum sample for determination of distemper titers.

34. The IgG is positive at 1:512; the IgM is negative.

35. Obtain radiographs of the abdomen.

35. The prostate is enlarged. All else is within normal limits.

36. Obtain radiographs of the thorax.

36. The right caudal lobar artery is enlarged and blunted. The right ventricle is mildly enlarged. All else is within normal limits.

37. Collect a blood sample for a Knott's exam.

37. The Knott's test is negative.

38. Perform a skin biopsy in the area of the swelling.

38. The biopsy is normal.

39. Perform an arthrocentesis on both carpi.

39. The cytology is normal.

40. Obtain radiographs of both carpi.

40. The joints appear normal.

41. Collect a urine sample for determination of protein:creatinine ratio.

41. The urine protein:creatinine ratio is 7:1.

42. Collect a serum sample for determination of parathyroid hormone (PTH) concentration.

42. The parathyroid hormone concentration is normal.

Go to Section D

Section D:

Considering the information you have gained so far, which further diagnostic procedures would you perform? *(Choose only the procedures you believe relevant to managing the case at this point.)*

43. Ejaculate the dog and collect a semen sample for cytology and culture.

43. No abnormalities are noted on cytology, and the culture is negative.

44. Collect a serum sample for *Blastomyces, Histoplasma,* and *Coccidioides* titers.

44. All titers are negative.

45. Obtain an echocardiographic examination.

45. On echocardiography the right ventricle and pulmonary artery is noted to be mildly enlarged.

46. Collect a serum sample for an occult heartworm test.

46. The test is positive.

47. Collect a serum sample for a *Brucella* card test.

47. The Brucella card test is negative.

48. Collect a serum sample for Rocky Mountain spotted fever titers.

48. The titer is positive at 1:512.

49. Measure the systolic blood pressure using a Doppler.

49. The systolic blood pressure is 110 mm Hg.

50. Perform an ultrasound-guided kidney biopsy.

50. The biopsy findings are consistent with glomerulonephritis.

51. Obtain serum samples for preprandial and postprandial bile acid determination.

51. The preprandial and postprandial bile acids are normal.

52. Perform an ultrasound-guided liver biopsy.

52. The liver biopsy is normal.

53. Collect a serum sample for measurement of trypsinlike immunoreactivity (TLI), folate, and cobalamin.

53. All results are within normal limits.

54. Perform endoscopy to obtain biopsies of the stomach and small intestine.

54. The biopsies are normal.

55. Obtain a serum sample for *Ehrlichia* titers.

55. The *Ehrlichia* titer is negative.

56. Obtain a serum sample for Lyme disease titers.

56. The Lyme disease titer is positive at 1:1024.

57. Obtain a serum sample for antinuclear antibody titer.

57. The antinuclear antibody titer is negative.

58. Obtain three blood samples 30 minutes apart for aerobic and anaerobic bacterial culture.

58. All cultures are negative.

59. Obtain a bone marrow aspirate for cytology.

59. The bone marrow is normal.

60. Perform a low dose dexamethasone suppression test.

60. Cortisol concentration in the predexamethasone sample is 2.5 µg/dl. At 4 hours post dexamethasone the cortisol is 1.5 µg/dl, and at 8 hours the cortisol is 1.0 µg/dl.

61. Obtain a serum sample for evaluation by immunoelectrophoresis.

61. The electrophoresis shows a polyclonal gammopathy.

Go to Section E

Section E:

Which course of action would you take? *(Choose only one.)*

62. Prescribe prednisone at 0.5 mg/kg b.i.d. for 4 weeks and recheck the dog at the end of treatment.

62. End of problem.

63. Prescribe doxycycline at 5 mg/kg b.i.d. for 21 days and recheck the dog at the end of treatment.

63. End of problem.

64. Administer caparsolate at 2.2 mg/kg b.i.d. IV for 2 days and recheck the dog in 1 week.

64. End of problem.

65. Place the dog on a high protein diet and recheck the dog in 2 weeks.

65. End of problem.

66. Place the dog on a low protein diet and recheck the dog in 2 weeks.

66. End of problem.

67. Prescribe furosemide at 2.2 mg/kg b.i.d. and recheck the dog in 1 week.

67. End of problem.

68. Recommend physical therapy for the dog, including massage and passive movement of the distal extremities.

68. End of problem.

69. Recommend that the dog be neutered.

69. End of problem.

END OF PROBLEM

Opening Scene:

A 5-year-old, 4.5 kg spayed female domestic shorthair cat is presented to your clinic with a chief complaint of difficulty breathing. The owners indicate that the cat has become more and more lethargic for the past 2 weeks and has not eaten in the past 2 days. The owners noted the cat to have rapid, shallow breathing today. Normally, the cat eats dry commercial cat food. It is current on all vaccinations (feline viral rhinotracheitis/calicivirus/pan-leukopenia virus and rabies). The cat is not in respiratory distress.

Go to Section A

Section A:

What questions would you ask the owner? (Choose only the questions you believe relevant to managing the case at this point.)

1. When did the respiratory difficulty start?

2. Is the cat an indoor or outdoor cat or both?

3. How is the cat's appetite normally?

4. Have you noticed any discharge from the eyes, nose, or vulva?

5. Has the cat had any coughing or sneezing?

6. Have you noticed any vomiting or diarrhea?

7. Have you noticed the cat to be lethargic before this illness?

8. Has your cat ever been ill before?

9. Has your cat had any previous trauma or surgery?

10. Has there been a change in water consumption?

11. Have you noticed any change in your cat's urinary habits?

12. Does your cat fight with other cats or dogs?

13. Do you have any other animals, and if so, are they healthy?

14. Is the cat on any medication(s)?

1. "About 3 days ago."

2. "Indoor and outdoor; stays indoor at night."

3. "Good, but it has been decreased for the last 2 weeks."

4. "No."

5. "No."

6. "No, but the cat urinates and defecates outside."

7. "Not until the past 2 weeks."

8. "No."

9. "The teeth were cleaned 3 months ago."

10. "No."

11. "No, but it urinates outside."

12. "Occasionally."

13. "I have one other cat and it is fine."

14. "No."

Go to Section B

Section B:

Which physical examination procedures would you perform at this time? *(Choose only the procedures you believe relevant to managing the case at this point.)*

15. Evaluate the cat's general appearance and hydration status.

15. Cat appears to have unkempt hair, is lethargic, and about 5% dehydrated.

16. Measure the rectal temperature.

16. 37.4°C.

17. Examine the oral cavity.

17. Normal.

18. Auscultate the heart and lungs; obtain a heart rate and respiratory rate.

18. The lung sounds are decreased on both sides. The respiratory pattern is rapid and shallow. The heart rate is rapid, but no murmur is heard. Heart rate is 180 beats per minute, respiration rate is 64 rpm.

19. Palpate for a femoral pulse.

19. Normal.

20. Palpate the peripheral lymph nodes.

20. Normal.

21. Palpate the abdomen.

21. Normal.

22. Test the chest for compressibility.

22. Decreased compressibility.

23. Check for pupillary light responses and perform a complete funduscopic exam.

23. Normal.

24. Examine the ears with an otoscope.

24. Ears are normal.

25. Examine the cat for evidence of trauma or external wounds.

25. No evidence of fighting.

26. Examine the cat's skin.

26. Increased shedding and scale.

Go to Section C

Section C:

Which diagnostic procedures would you perform at this time? *(Choose only the procedures you believe relevant to managing the case at this point.)*

27. Collect a blood sample for a complete blood count.

27. The complete blood count results show the following:
Nucleated cells = 38,300/mm^3
Bands = 10,300/mm^3
Neutrophils = 26,800/mm^3
Lymphocytes = 400/mm^3
Monocytes = 800/mm^3
Notes = marked toxic neutrophils
Plasma protein = 8.7 g/dl
RBC = 5.65 million/mm^3
Hemoglobin = 9.3 g/dl

PCV = 28%
MCV = 50 fl
MCHC = 33 g/dl
Platelets = adequate

28. Collect a urine sample for urinalysis.

28. The urinalysis is as follows:
specific gravity = 1.054
pH = 7.0
Blood = negative
Ketones = negative
Glucose = negative
Protein = negative
Bilirubin = negative
No sediment analysis available.

29. Collect a blood sample for FeLV, FIV, and FIP serology.

29. FeLV negative for p27 antigen by ELISA; FIV negative for antibodies by ELISA; FIP 1:100 by IFA.

30. Radiograph the chest.

30. Marked pleural effusion bilaterally. Nothing else can be determined due to the fluid present.

31. Perform a diagnostic thoracocentesis from the left side and submit a sample of any fluid obtained for cytology.

31. 150 ml of brown flocculent material with small yellow granules is removed. On cytology, there are many neutrophils and some macrophages. There are many intracellular and extracellular filamentous bacteria. Conclusion: septic, suppurative inflammation of bacterial cause.

32. Perform a diagnostic thoracocentesis from the right side and submit a sample of any fluid obtained for cytology.

32. 120 ml of brown flocculent material with small yellow granules is removed. On cytology, there are many neutrophils and some macrophages. There are many intracellular and extracellular filamentous bacteria. Conclusion: septic, suppurative inflammation of bacterial cause.

33. Collect a blood sample for a biochemistry profile.

33. The biochemistry profile is as follows:
Glucose = 97 mg/dl
BUN = 27 mg/dl
Creatinine = 1.1 mg/dl
Phosphate = 5.8 mg/dl
Calcium = 8.3 mg/dl
Total protein = 8.6 g/dl
Albumin = 2.4 g/dl
Globulin = 6.2 g/dl
Cholesterol = 98 mg/dl
Total bilirubin = 0.3 mg/dl
ALP = 4 IU/L
ALT = 13 IU/L
AST = 32 IU/L
GGT = 2 IU/L
Sodium = 147 mEq/L
Potassium = 4.5 mEq/L
Chloride = 109 mEq/L
Total CO_2 = 10.7 mEq/L
Anion gap = 32

34. Collect a blood sample for *Toxoplasma* serology.

34. IgM negative, IgG negative.

35. Perform an orotracheal wash and submit a sample for cytology.

35. Few epithelial cells seen.

36. Perform a diagnostic peritoneal lavage and submit a sample for cytology.

36. Few cells seen.

37. Perform a gastrointestinal radiographic contrast procedure.

37. Normal.

38. Collect a blood sample for triiodothyronine (T_3) and thyroxine (T_4) levels.

38. Triiodothyronine (T_3) 0.6 ng/ml; thyroxine (T_4) 1.2 µg/dl.

Go to Section D

Section D:

Based on what you know so far, which treatments or further diagnostics would you choose at this time? *(Choose only the procedures you believe relevant to managing the case at this point.)*

39. Perform an acid-fast stain on the chest fluid.

39. Bacteria are acid-fast negative.

40. Perform a gram stain on the chest fluid.

40. Gram positive bacteria.

41. Submit a sample from thoracocentesis for aerobic culture and antibiotic sensitivity.

41. No growth.

42. Submit a sample from thoracocentesis for anaerobic culture.

42. Cultured in heavy growth *Actinomyces* spp.

43. Radiograph the chest after thoracocentesis.

43. Small amount of pleural effusion noted. No masses or signs of pneumonia evident.

44. Lavage the chest with lactated Ringer's solution warmed to body temperature.

44. Done. A lot of floculent material is drained.

45. Administer IV fluids.

45. Done.

46. Exploratory surgery of the thorax.

46. Fibrinous pleuritis with lung retraction noted; no source of bacterial infection identified (i.e. foreign body, abscess, etc.).

47. Perform a fecal flotation and Baerman procedure to check for lung parasites.

47. Negative for parasites.

48. Perform bilateral tube thoracostomy.

48. Done.

49. Radiograph the chest after thoracostomy tube placement.

49. Tube placement is good bilaterally. Very mild pneumothorax and mild pleural effusion are present. No masses or evidence of pneumonia are seen.

50. Start sodium ampicillin IV at 22 mg/kg q.i.d.   50. Done.

51. Start gentamicin sulfate IV at 3 mg/kg t.i.d.   51. Done.

52. Perform daily bilateral thoracocentesis.   52. Done.

Go to Section E

Section E:

Which course of action would you take? (Choose only one.)

53. Advise the owner the prognosis is poor and recommend euthanasia.   53. End of problem.

54. Advise the owner the prognosis is guarded, but with time and intensive care, the cat may recover.   54. End of problem.

55. Advise the owner that there is no reason the cat cannot be managed at home with oral antibiotics.   55. End of problem.

56. Advise the owner that the cat has an excellent prognosis.   56. End of problem.

57. Advise the owner to start looking for a new cat.   57. End of problem.

END OF PROBLEM

Opening Scene:

An owner presents a 4.5 kg, 2-year-old male intact domestic shorthair cat to you with a chief complaint of an open, oozing sore on the left side of the cat's nose. The owner has noticed the lesion for about 2 weeks, but it has progressively increased in size. The cat is current on all vaccinations (feline viral rhinotracheitis/calicivirus/panleukopenia virus and rabies). The cat's diet consists of a commercial dry food.

Go to Section A

Section A:

What questions would you ask the owner? *(Choose only the questions you believe relevant to managing the case at this point.)*

1. How long has the lesion been apparent?

2. Is the cat an indoor or outdoor cat or both?

3. Does the lesion appear to bother the cat (e.g., does it scratch at the lesion)?

4. Does the cat get involved in fights?

5. Have you noticed any vomiting or diarrhea?

6. Have you noticed any coughing or sneezing?

7. Does the cat appear to see normally?

8. Have you noticed any change in the cat's water consumption?

9. How is the cat's appetite?

10. Is the cat on any medication(s)?

11. Has the cat had any previous illness, injury, or surgery?

12. Do you have any other pets, and if so, are they healthy?

13. Have you noticed any discharge from the eyes or nose?

1. "About 2 weeks ago."

2. "Outdoor."

3. "The cat does not scratch or paw at the lesion."

4. "Yes."

5. "No."

6. "Some mild sneezing."

7. "Yes."

8. "The water consumption seems to be a little decreased if anything."

9. "Poor."

10. "No."

11. "No."

12. "No, we have no other pets."

13. "No."

Go to Section B

Section B:

Which physical examination procedures would you perform at this time? *(Choose only the procedures you believe relevant to managing the case at this point.)*

14. Evaluate the cat's general appearance and hydration status.

    14. Cat appears to be about 5% dehydrated with thin, unkempt hair.

15. Measure the rectal temperature.

    15. 39.9°C.

16. Auscultate the chest for heart and lung sounds. Determine heart and respiratory rates.

    16. The heart and lung sounds are normal. The heart rate is 174 beats per minute, and the respiratory rate is 32 rpm.

17. Palpate each rear limb to assess the femoral pulse.

    17. Normal.

18. Closely examine the lesion.

    18. The lesion is foul smelling, crusting on the edges, with a necrotic-looking center. It is about 1 cm by 0.5 cm in size. Some exudate is crusted on the cat's fur where the lesion drains.

19. Closely examine the cat for any other skin lesions.

    19. No other lesions noted.

20. Palpate all peripheral lymph nodes.

    20. Both submandibular lymph nodes are slightly large.

21. Examine the oral cavity.

    21. Normal.

22. Assess the pupillary light responses.

    22. Normal.

23. Examine the ears with an otoscope.

    23. Normal.

24. Perform a funduscopic examination.

    24. Normal.

25. Express urine from the cat's bladder.

    25. Normal.

26. Assess spinal and postural reflexes, gait, and proprioception.

    26. Normal.

Go to Section C

Section C:

Which diagnostic or therapeutic procedures would you perform at this time? *(Choose only the procedures you believe relevant to managing the case at this point.)*

27. Place the cat on cephalexin 22 mg/kg t.i.d. PO for 3 weeks and send it home.

    27. Done. End of problem.

28. Collect blood for a complete blood count.

28. The complete blood count results show the following:
Nucleated cells = 30,600/μl
Bands = 200/mm^3
Neutrophils = 24,300/mm^3
Lymphocytes = 5900/mm^3
Monocytes = 1200/mm^3
Plasma protein = 8.7 g/dl
RBC = 8.76 million/mm^3
Hemoglobin = 12.7 g/dl
PCV = 42%
MCV = 48 fl
MCHC = 30 g/dl
Platelets = adequate

29. Collect blood for a biochemistry panel.

29. The biochemistry profile is as follows:
Glucose = 100 mg/dl
BUN = 24 mg/dl
Creatinine = 0.9 mg/dl
Phosphate = 4.5 mg/dl
Calcium = 8.4 mg/dl
Total protein = 9.1 g/dl
Albumin = 4.2 g/dl
Globulin = 4.9 g/dl
Cholesterol = 78 mg/dl
Total bilirubin = 0.1 mg/dl
ALP = 10 IU/L
ALT = 45 IU/L
AST = 15 IU/L
GGT = 1 IU/L
Sodium = 151 mEq/L
Potassium = 4.0 mEq/L
Chloride = 115 mEq/L
Total CO2 = 15 mEq/L
Anion gap = 25

30. Collect urine by cystocentesis for a urinalysis.

30. The urinalysis results are as follows:
specific gravity = 1.054
pH = 7.0
Blood = negative
Ketones = negative
Glucose = negative
Protein = negative
Bilirubin = negative
No sediment analysis available.

31. Collect blood for FeLV and FIV serology.

31. FeLV p27 antigen ELISA negative; FIV antibody ELISA negative.

32. Collect blood for a *Cryptococcus* antigen test.

32. *Cryptococcus* antigen latex agglutination negative.

33. Collect blood for triiodothyronine (T$_3$) and thyroxine (T$_4$) levels.

33. Triiodothyronine (T$_3$) 0.6 ng/ml; Thyroxine (T$_4$) 1.7 μg/dl.

34. Make impression smears of the facial lesion, stain with a Wright's stain, and examine cytologically.

34. Wright-Giemsa stain. Many macrophages and degenerate neutrophils are seen. Within some macrophages and extracellular are multiple cigar-shaped pleomorphic yeast consistent with *Sporothrix schenckii.*

35. Radiograph the chest.

35. Normal.

36. Pluck hairs to culture for dermatophytes.

36. Done. Culture will be ready in 10 days.

37. Skin scrape near the affected area for mites.

37. No mites seen.

38. Perform a biopsy of the affected area.

38. Multiple areas of necrosis with many inflammatory cells. Many cigar-shaped pleomorphic yeast consistent with *Sporothrix schenckii.*

39. Anesthetize the cat and do skull radiographs.

39. Increased soft tissue density on the left side of the nose. No bony lesions evident.

40. Anesthetize the cat and do rhinoscopy with culture and biopsy.

40. No abnormalities seen. Histopathologically normal. Medium growth of *Pasteurella* spp.

41. Aspirate the submandibular lymph nodes and perform cytology.

41. Cytology consistent with reactive lymph node.

Go to Section D

Section D:

Which therapeutic procedures would you perform? *(Select only the therapies you believe relevant to managing the case at this point.)*

42. Place the cat on cephalexin 22 mg/kg PO t.i.d. and send it home.

42. Done.

43. Start treatment with potassium iodide at 20 mg/kg PO b.i.d.

43. Done.

44. Start treatment with itraconazole 5 mg/kg PO b.i.d.

44. Done.

45. Start treatment with ketoconazole 5 mg/kg PO b.i.d.

45. Done.

46. Start treatment with enrofloxacin 2.5 mg/kg PO b.i.d.

46. Done.

47. Completely excise the lesion surgically.

47. Completed.

48. Start the cat on IV lactated Ringer's solution.

48. Done. Cat feels better and starts eating.

49. Observe the cat in your hospital overnight.

49. Done. Cat feels better and starts eating after fluid therapy.

50. Start prednisone at 1 mg/kg daily PO.

50. Done.

Section E:

Which course of action would you take on advising the owner? *(Choose only two.)*

51. Advise the owner that in cats this disease never disseminates, so recovery should be rapid.

51. Done.

52. Advise the owner that this disease can disseminate in cats and it does require long-term therapy.

52. Done.

53. Advise the owners of the public health significance of this organism.

53. Done.

54. Advise the owner that there is no risk of transmission of this organism from cats to people.

54. Done.

55. Recommend euthanasia based on the public health risk and poor prognosis.

55. Done.

56. Advise the owner that this disease is usually transmitted from children to their pets.

56. Done.

END OF PROBLEM

Opening Scene:

You are in a six-person small animal practice in El Paso, Texas (far west Texas, on the New Mexico and Mexico border). A client presents a 20 kg, 3-year-old, intact male Labrador retriever for lameness of the right forelimb. The lameness has been present for 2 months. The dog is current on all vaccinations (distemper/hepatitis/parvovirus/parainfluenza, rabies). The dog eats a commercial, good quality dry dog food.

Go to Section A

Section A:

What questions would you ask the owner? (*Choose only the questions you believe relevant to managing the case at this point.*)

1. Does the lameness come and go or is the severity of the lameness staying the same or progressively getting worse?

   1. "It is getting worse."

2. Has the dog had any prior illness?

   2. "No."

3. Is the dog an indoor or outdoor dog or both?

   3. "Both. We live on a ranch and the dog goes with me when I ride to check the cattle."

4. How is the dog's appetite?

   4. "Poor lately."

5. Have you noticed any coughing or sneezing?

   5. "About 9 to 10 months ago, the dog seemed to cough a good deal, but he got better."

6. Have you noticed any discharge from the eyes or nose?

   6. "No."

7. Has there been any vomiting or diarrhea?

   7. "No."

8. Have you noticed any vision problems?

   8. "No."

9. Does the leg seem painful when you touch it?

   9. "Yes, when I touch it, he gets apprehensive."

10. Has there been any change in water consumption?

    10. "No."

11. Has there been any change in urinary habits?

    11. "No."

12. Is the dog on any medication(s)?

    12. "Aspirin for his lameness, one 325 mg buffered aspirin twice daily."

13. Has the dog been lame before?

    13. "No."

14. Has the dog been injured or had any surgery before?

    14. "No."

15. Has the dog had any behavioral changes or seizures?

    15. "No."

Go to Section B

Section B:

Which physical examination procedures would you perform at this time? *(Choose only the procedures you believe relevant to managing the case at this point.)*

16. Evaluate the dog's general appearance and hydration status.

16. The dog is slightly dehydrated (about 5%); he seems thin and is depressed.

17. Measure a rectal temperature.

17. 38.9°C.

18. Auscultate the heart and lungs.

18. Normal.

19. Determine a heart rate and respiration rate.

19. The heart rate is 84 beats per minute; respiratory rate is 18 per minute.

20. Palpate the femoral pulses.

20. Normal.

21. Evaluate the dog's peripheral lymph nodes.

21. Enlarged right axillary lymph node.

22. Do a complete eye exam including a funduscopic exam.

22. Normal.

23. Palpate the dog's abdomen.

23. Normal.

24. Perform a complete orthopedic evaluation.

24. The right distal radius is warm to the touch, swollen, and painful upon deep palpation.

25. Perform a rectal exam.

25. Normal.

26. Examine the ears with an otoscope.

26. Normal.

27. Perform a complete neurological examination.

27. Normal.

28. Thoroughly evaluate the skin for presence of lesions.

28. No lesions found.

Go to Section C

Section C:

Which diagnostic tests would you perform at this time? *(Choose only the procedures you believe relevant to managing the case at this point.)*

29. Collect a blood sample for a complete blood count.

29. The complete blood count results show the following:
WBC = 30,600/mm^3
Bands = 500/mm^3
Neutrophils = 25,400/mm^3
Lymphocytes = 3600/mm^3
Monocytes = 1600/mm^3
Plasma protein = 8.7 g/dl
RBC = 4.77 million/mm^3
Hemoglobin = 10.8 g/dl

PCV = 32%
MCV = 67 fl
MCHC = 34 g/dl
Platelets = 352,000/mm^3

30. Collect a blood sample for a biochemistry panel.

30. The biochemistry panel results are as follows:
Glucose = 101 mg/dl
BUN = 11 mg/dl
Creatinine = 0.6 mg/dl
Phosphate = 5.0 mg/dl
Calcium = 8.0 mg/dl
Total protein = 8.8 g/dl
Albumin = 2.5 g/dl
Globulin = 6.3 g/dl
Cholesterol = 130 mg/dl
Total bilirubin = 0.2 mg/dl
ALP = 121 IU/L
ALT = 56 IU/L
AST = 32 IU/L
GGT = 3 IU/L
Sodium = 146 mEq/L
Potassium = 4.1 mEq/L
Chloride = 110 mEq/L
Total CO2= 24 mEq/L
Anion gap = 12

31. Collect urine by cystocentesis for a urinalysis.

31. Urinalysis results are as follows:
Specific gravity = 1.038
pH = 7.0
Blood = negative
Ketones = negative
Glucose = negative
Protein = negative
Bilirubin = 1+
No sediment analysis available.

32. Collect blood for a triiodothyronine (T$_3$) and thyroxine (T$_4$) level.

32. Triiodothyronine (T$_3$) 1.0 ng/ml; thyroxine (T$_4$) 2.02 µg/dl.

33. Radiograph the chest.

33. No abnormalities seen.

34. Radiograph the right distal radius.

34. Periosteal new bone formation and osteolysis of the distal right radius, consistent with neoplasia or osteomyelitis.

35. Perform a joint tap of the right carpus.

35. Cannot get fluid.

36. Aspirate the right axillary lymph node and evaluate cytologically.

36. Pyogranulomatous inflammation. No organisms or etiology seen.

37. Collect blood for histoplasmosis, blastomycosis, and coccidioidomycosis antibody titers, and cryptococcoses antigen titers.

37. *Histoplasma* titer negative;
Blastomyces titer negative;
Coccidioides titer 1:32;
Cryptococcus antigen titer negative.

38. Radiograph the abdomen.

38. Normal.

39. Perform a prostatic wash.

39. Normal.

40. Perform a cerebrospinal fluid tap.

40. Normal.

41. Collect blood for *Neospora* and *Toxoplasma* antibody titers.

41. *Toxoplasma* IgM and IgG negative; *Neospora* IgM negative.

Go to Section D

Section D:

Based on the information you have gathered so far, which additional diagnostics and/or therapeutics would you perform? *(Choose only the procedures you believe relevant to managing the case at this time.)*

42. Amputate the right forelimb.

42. Done. End of problem.

43. Amputate the right forelimb and submit a sample of the lesion for histopathology.

43. Done.

44. Perform a vitreal tap for cytology on both eyes.

44. Done.

45. Anesthetize the patient and biopsy the lesion in the right forelimb.

45. Done.

46. Perform an arthrocentesis on the right carpus for cytological examination and aerobic and anaerobic bacterial culture and antibiotic sensitivity.

46. Negative.

47. Start treatment with clindamycin 10 mg/kg PO b.i.d.

47. Done. End of problem.

48. Perform cytology on impression smears from your biopsy.

48. Done. Many neutrophils present and few large fungal spherules with endospores consistent with *Coccidioides immitis*.

49. Perform a bone biopsy on the anesthetized dog and submit the biopsy for histopathology with special stains for fungi.

49. Done. Periosteal new bone growth with large numbers of inflammatory cells. Increased osteoclastic activity. Few large fungal spherules with endospores surrounded by many neutrophils are noted. Severe osteomyelitis consistent with coccidioidomycosis.

Go to Section E

Section E:

Based on what you know now, what treatment would you perform? *(Choose only one.)*

50. Start treatment with itraconazole at 5 mg/kg PO b.i.d.

50. Done. End of problem.

51. Start treatment with potassium iodide at 20 mg/kg PO b.i.d.

51. Done. End of problem.

52. Start treatment with cisplatin 70 mg/m^2 IV once every 3 weeks.

52. Done. End of problem.

53. Amputate the limb.

53. Done. End of problem.

54. Amputate the limb and start itraconazole at 5 mg/kg PO b.i.d.

54. Done. End of problem.

55. Amputate the limb and start treatment with cisplatin 70 mg/m^2 IV once every 3 weeks.

55. Done. End of problem.

END OF PROBLEM

Opening Scene:

It is a snowy December morning in the Midwestern United States. You have a message to call a client regarding his 10-foot male Burmese python, *Python molorus bivittatus,* with a suspected respiratory infection.

Go to Section A

Section A:

What questions would you like to ask the owner? *(Choose only the questions you believe relevant to managing the case at this point.)*

1. What makes you think the snake has a respiratory problem?

1. "He is wheezing."

2. Is there any discharge from the snake's nares?

2. "No, except when the snake is drinking."

3. Have you heard any gurgling respiratory sounds?

3. "No."

4. What sort of cage is the snake kept in?

4. We have a 100 gallon aquarium with a fitted top.

5. Is the snake opaque or getting ready to shed?

5. "Yes, the snake has been opaque for the last week. 5 days ago the eyes were blue and 2 days ago, the snake's eyes cleared. This morning the snake shed his skin."

6. Has the snake been chilled at all?

6. "The snake is in a cage that gets no colder than 75°F at night and warms to 85°F to 90°F during the day."

7. How is the cage heated?

7. "The room is heated to 75°F with an electric oil-filled radiator. Spot heat is supplied under one end of the cage with a heating pad and a 75 watt light bulb outside and above the cage."

8. Does the snake exhibit open mouth breathing?

8. "No."

9. Is the snake still eating?

9. "Yes, it ate a rabbit last week before shedding. He eats one rabbit about every 3 to 6 weeks usually."

10. Is the snake gravid?

10. "No, he is a male."

11. Have you been handling the snake more than usual?

11. "No, you told me not to handle him when he was shedding."

Go to Section B

Section B:

What recommendations would you make to the owner? *(Choose only those responses that you believe relevant to managing the case at this point).*

12. Bring the snake in a cloth bag to the clinic so it can be examined.

12. Done.

13. Wait until the weather warms up and examine the snake then.

13. Done.

Go to Section C

Section C:

What physical examination procedures would you perform at this time? *(Choose only those procedures you believe relevant to managing the case at this point.)*

14. Obtain a body weight.

14. 44 kg.

15. Examine the snake's head.

15. The periocular and gular areas are filled with mites.

16. Examine the oral cavity.

16. The mouth is pale pink. There are no petechial hemorrhages nor is a glottal discharge present.

17. Auscultate the area over the nares with the open bell of the stethoscope.

17. Inspiration is silent and expiration is audible with no evidence of rales or gurgles.

18. Auscultate the lungs.

18. Inspiration is silent and expiration is audible, with no rales or gurgles; however, the skin makes a lot of noise rubbing against the stethoscope.

19. Auscultate the lungs after placing a damp paper towel over the skin.

19. The lung sounds are normal.

20. Observe the snake at rest.

20. The snake is coiled with the head resting on one coil. The tongue flicks periodically.

21. Palpate the entire length of the snake.

21. No abnormalities noted, but difficult to perform.

22. Examine the cloaca.

22. No significant findings, although small spurs are noted.

23. Determine the sex of the snake.

23. The snake probes less than three subcaudals indicating it is a female. The owner is pleasantly surprised.

Go to Section D

Section D:

What diagnostic/therapeutic procedures would you like to perform? *(Choose only those procedures and therapies that are relevant to managing the case at this point.)*

24. Obtain blood for a complete blood count.

24. The complete blood count results show the following:
RBC = 1.4 million/mm^3
WBC = 7200/mm^3
Heterophils = 2900/mm^3
Azurophils = 1100/mm^3
Lymphocytes = 3000/mm^3
Monocytes = 0/mm^3
Eosinophils = 0/mm^3
Basophils = 200/mm^3

25. Obtain blood for a plasma chemistry analysis.

25. The plasma chemistry analysis results are as follows:
Calcium = 10.2 mg/dl
Phosphorus = 5.5 mg/dl
Total protein = 7.5 g/dl
AST = 25 IU/l
BUN = 1.8 mg/dl
Creatinine <0.1 mg/dl
Uric acid = 4.6 mg/dl
Glucose = 55 mg/dl
Sodium = 146 mEq/L
Potassium = 3.5 mEq/L

26. Obtain radiographs of the anterior quarter, including the head.

26. Normal.

27. Obtain radiographs of the middle anterior quarter of the snake.

27. Normal.

28. Obtain radiographs of the middle posterior quarter of the snake.

28. Normal.

29. Obtain radiographs of the caudal quarter of the snake including the tail.

29. Normal.

30. Prescribe bactericidal antibiotics for 3 weeks and schedule a recheck examination in 1 week.

30. Done.

31. Perform a stomach wash for cytological examination.

31. No significant findings.

32. Administer a multivitamin injection and schedule a recheck examination in 1 week.

32. Done.

33. Collect feces for fecal examination.

33. Negative.

34. Collect oral samples for aerobic and anaerobic bacterial culture and antibiotic sensitivity.

34. Light growth of coagulase-negative *Staphylococcus* spp., *Pseudomonas aeruginosa*, and *Corynebacterium* spp., sensitive to most antibiotics.

35. Collect glottal sample for aerobic and anaerobic bacterial cultures and antibiotic sensitivity.

35. Light growth of *Providencia rettgeri*, coagulase-negative *Staphylococcus* spp., *Pseudomonas aeruginosa*, sensitive to most antibiotics.

36. Collect tracheal samples for aerobic bacterial culture and antibiotic sensitivity.

36. Light growth of *Providencia rettgeri*, coagulase-negative *Staphylococcus* spp., sensitive to most antibiotics.

37. Anesthetize the snake and perform endoscopy of the respiratory tract.

37. No abnormal findings.

Go to Section E

Section E:

Considering the information you have gained so far, what therapeutic recommendations would you make? (*Choose only those therapies that you believe relevant to managing the case at this time.*)

38. Prescribe a 3 week course of enrofloxacin at a dose of 5 mg/kg IM every 48 hours.

38. End of problem.

39. Prescribe a 3 week course of amikacin at a dose of 5 mg/kg IM (loading dose) followed by 2.5 mg/kg IM every 72 hours.

39. End of problem.

40. Prescribe fenbendazole for roundworms at a dose of 50 mg/kg via gavage every 2 weeks for four treatments.

40. End of problem.

41. Treat the cage and snake with 1% trichlorfon spray once weekly for three treatments.

41. The client is thankful to be rid of the mites. End of problem.

42. Advise the client that antibiotics are not necessary since the snake does not appear to have a respiratory infection at this time.

42. Correct. End of problem.

43. Dip the snake in olive oil and clean the cage thoroughly.

43. The mites recur because the cage wasn't treated. End of problem.

44. Advise the owner to raise the cage temperature by 10°F for 2 weeks.

44. The snake shows signs of heat stress. End of problem.

45. Prescribe ivermectin at a dose of 0.2 mg/kg IM every 2 weeks for 14 treatments.

45. The mites recur because the cage wasn't treated. End of problem.

END OF PROBLEM

Opening Scene:

It is a warm summer afternoon in the Midwestern United States. A young mother with two young children present their 3-year-old iguana, *Iguana iguana,* which she purchased 3 months ago from a private owner. She is concerned that the iguana has been eating very little lately. The iguana weighs 1 kg.

Go to Section A

Section A:

What questions would you like to ask the owner? (*Choose only the questions you believe relevant to managing the case at this point.*)

1. What do you normally feed your iguana?

2. Do you supplement the diet with vitamins?

3. Do you supplement the diet with calcium?

4. What is the minimum cage temperature at night and the maximum cage temperature during the day?

5. Is there a thermometer for accurate measurement?

6. Does the iguana have access to ultraviolet lights?

7. What type of lights do you have for the cage?

8. Does the iguana have access to unfiltered sunlight?

9. Besides eating less, is your iguana acting abnormal in any other ways?

10. Does your iguana exhibit any breathing difficulties?

11. Does your iguana have any difficulty walking?

12. How often do you clean the cage?

---

1. "Vegetables and fruits."

2. "Yes, she gets a sprinkling of multivitamins on her food."

3. "The multivitamins contain calcium."

4. "The cage gets down to 70°F at night and warms to 80°F to 85°F during the day."

5. "No, I'm just guessing at the temperature."

6. "Yes."

7. "They are regular aquarium lights."

8. "I put her in front of the window to bask, but it's been too cold to put her outside."

9. "She seems restless and also she seems to be trying to dig out of her cage."

10. "No."

11. "I can't really tell for sure."

12. "Once a week."

Section B:

What physical examination procedures would you perform at this time? *(Choose only those procedures you believe relevant to managing the case at this point.)*

13. Observe the iguana walking.

13. She drags her pelvis and tail along the ground and seems to have pain in the right front leg.

14. Examine the oral cavity.

14. The mucous membranes are pale pink. The tip of the tongue is bifurcated and bright red.

15. Palpate the mandible and maxillae.

15. Both bones are more pliable than normal.

16. Examine the vertebral column for lordosis, kyphosis, or scoliosis.

16. None present.

17. Auscultate the lungs after placing a damp paper towel over the skin.

17. Normal.

18. Note the overall body condition.

18. Overall body condition is good; however, coelom seems very full.

19. Palpate the entire length of the tail.

19. Normal.

20. Examine the cloaca.

20. Normal.

21. Determine the sex of the iguana.

21. Small femoral pores, jowls, and dorsal spinous crest scales suggest it is a female.

22. Throw the iguana in the air for a short distance to observe how well the iguana uses its legs.

22. Done. The left femur fractures; the client and patient are very distraught.

23. Palpate the abdomen.

23. The abdomen feels full, but it is difficult to discern why.

24. Palpate the bones and muscles of the limbs.

24. All limbs are normal except the right humerus, which is thickened and unstable.

25. Examine the skin.

25. Normal.

26. Examine the eyes and nares.

26. Normal.

Go to Section C

Section C:

What diagnostic/therapeutic procedures would you like to perform? *(Choose only those procedures/therapies that you believe relevant to managing the case at this point.)*

27. Obtain blood for a complete blood count.

27. The complete blood count results show the following:
RBC = 1.2 million/mm^3
WBC = 6500/mm^3

Heterophils = 2300/mm^3
Azurophils = 1100/mm^3
Lymphocytes = 2700/mm^3
Monocytes = 60/mm^3
Eosinophils = 130/mm^3
Basophils = 210/mm^3

28. Obtain blood for a plasma chemistry analysis.

28. The results of the plasma chemistry analysis show the following:
Calcium = 6.3 mg/dl
Phosphorus = 6.2 mg/dl
Total protein = 7.5 g/dl
Albumin = 3.1 g/dl
AST = 28 IU/L
ALT = 20 IU/L
Uric acid = 2.6 mg/dl
Glucose = 105 mg/dl
Sodium = 155 mEq/L
Potassium = 2.7 mEq/L

29. Obtain radiographs of the whole body.

29. Overall bone density is reduced, particularly in the pelvis and vertebral processes. There is a midshaft humeral fracture. Partial outlines of numerous round structures 2 cm in diameter are seen in the caudal coelom.

30. Instruct the owner to feed the iguana a more balanced diet, provide full spectrum ultraviolet lights, and administer calcium supplements instead of a multivitamin. Schedule a recheck examination in 2 weeks.

30. Done. The iguana returns in much worse shape and the owner is very upset.

31. Administer barium orally and radiograph the iguana.

31. The stomach is pushed cranially but is otherwise normal.

32. Perform an abdominocentesis.

32. Done. You aspirate 0.5 ml of a thick yellow fluid.

33. Collect feces for fecal examination.

33. Positive for pinworms *(Oxyuris).*

34. Collect cloacal samples for a gram stain and cytology.

34. Done. Predominately gram-negative organisms seen.

Go to Section D

Section D:

Considering the information you have gained so far, what are the iguana's primary problems? *(Choose only those problems that are relevant to the case at this point.)*

35. Bacterial coelomitis (peritonitis).

35. Response noted.

36. Endoparasitism.

36. Response noted.

37. Retained follicles/eggs.

37. Response noted.

38. Infectious stomatitis.

39. Gastrointestinal gram-negative bacterial overgrowth.

40. Anorexia.

41. Metabolic bone disease.

38. Response noted.

39. Response noted.

40. Response noted.

41. Response noted.

Go to Section E

Section E:

Considering the information you have gained so far, what therapeutic recommendations would you make? *(Choose only those therapies that you believe relevant to managing the case at this point.)*

42. Prescribe broad spectrum oral antibiotics for 3 weeks.

42. Done. No improvement.

43. Prescribe broad spectrum intramuscular bacteriocidal antibiotics for 3 weeks.

43. Done. No improvement.

44. Prescribe fenbendazole at a dose of 50 mg/kg via gavage every 2 weeks for four treatments.

44. Done. No improvement.

45. Flush mouth and tongue daily with dilute chlorhexidine.

45. Done. No improvement.

46. Instruct the owner to feed a more balanced diet, provide full spectrum ultraviolet light, and administer calcium supplements instead of a multivitamin. Schedule a recheck examination in 2 weeks.

46. Done. The iguana returns in worse condition and the owner is very upset.

47. Administer 50 IU salmon calcitonin IM; repeat in 1 week.

47. Done. The iguana's condition deteriorates into a hypocalcemic tetany.

48. Administer 1 ml/kg calcium glibionate (Neocalglucon) PO twice daily for 1 to 3 months.

48. Done. The iguana's attitude improves but the anorexia continues.

49. Schedule the iguana for surgery to remove the ovaries and follicles or eggs in the next few weeks.

49. Done. The iguana makes a full recovery.

50. Set up a nest area for the iguana.

50. Done. The iguana lays 37 eggs.

51. Perform exploratory surgery of coelom and aerobic/anaerobic bacterial culture of yellowish material in the coelom.

51. Done. No abnormal findings. No growth on bacterial culture.

Go to Section F

Section F:

Considering the information you have gained so far, what recommendations regarding husbandry would you give the owner? *(Choose only those recommendations that you believe relevant to managing the case at this point.)*

52. Use a calcium supplement instead of a multivitamin on a daily basis.

52. Correct. End of problem.

53. Get rid of the iguana because she'll be chronically ill.

53. End of problem.

54. Provide full spectrum ultraviolet light or outdoor sunlight exposure on a regular basis.

54. Correct. End of problem.

55. Feed a well-balanced diet.

55. Correct. End of problem.

56. Do not allow the iguana free run of the house.

56. Correct. This is especially important since the owner has young children and iguanas carry *Salmonella*. End of problem.

57. Discuss salmonellosis.

57. Correct. This is especially important since the owner has young children and iguanas carry *Salmonella*. End of problem.

END OF PROBLEM

Opening Scene:

A 4½-year-old female ferret is brought to you one August morning at your small animal/exotic pet practice in the midwestern United States. The owner complains that the ferret has been losing hair and has a swollen vulva. Vaccinations, including rabies and canine distemper, are up to date.

Go to Section A

Section A:

What questions would you like to ask the owner? (*Choose only the questions you believe relevant to managing the case at this point.*)

1. What do you normally feed your ferret?

1. "She eats a high quality cat food supplemented with feline hairball laxative twice a week."

2. How long have you noticed the hair loss?

2. "It began in February and has gotten progressively worse."

3. Does the ferret seem itchy?

3. "No, except she does scratch at her ears."

4. Where on the body did the hair loss start?

4. "It started at the base of the tail and spread forward towards the head."

5. Is it an indoor or an outdoor ferret?

5. "The "it" is a she and she is an exclusively indoor ferret."

6. Has there been any change in her activity level?

6. "No."

7. Has there been any change in her thirst?

7. "No."

8. How often do you bathe your ferret?

8. "Once every 2 weeks with a high quality dog shampoo."

9. Is your ferret spayed?

9. "Yes, she was spayed and descented before we got her."

10. Has there been any vaginal discharge?

10. "Occasionally."

11. When was her last heat?

11. "No, she was spayed."

12. Is there any possibility of trauma?

12. "No."

Go to Section B

Section B:

What physical examination procedures would you perform at this time? (*Choose only those procedures you believe relevant to managing the case at this point.*)

13. Measure the rectal temperature.

13. 38.5°C.

14. Place a small cat muzzle on the ferret before further examination.

14. The ferret instantly removes the muzzle much to your chagrin and the owner's delight.

15. Hold the ferret by its scruff and examine the oral cavity when it opens its mouth.

15. Slight dental tartar but otherwise normal oral cavity.

16. Gently compress the anterior thorax.

16. Slight compressibility, within normal limits.

17. Palpate the abdomen.

17. No abnormalities detected.

18. Examine the skin in the areas of hair loss.

18. There is a bilaterally symmetrical alopecia beginning over the caudal head and neck and continuing over the dorsal thorax and lumbosacral area. The skin is thin but no inflammatory lesions or petechia are noted.

19. Examine the ears with an otoscope.

19. There is a moderate amount of dry, crusty exudate within the ear canals. Two small black tattoos are noted on the back of the right ear indicating the ferret has been neutered and descented.

20. Auscultate the heart and lungs.

20. Normal auscultation with sinus arrhythmia.

21. Examine the vulva.

21. The vulva is swollen and a clear, mucoid discharge is noted.

22. Obtain a body weight.

22. 614 g.

23. Palpate the peripheral lymph nodes.

23. Normal.

Go to Section C

Section C:

What diagnostic/therapeutic procedures would you like to perform? (*Choose only those procedures/therapies that are relevant to managing the case at this point.*)

24. Obtain blood from the jugular vein for a complete blood count.

24. The complete blood count results show the following:
PCV = 42%
Hemoglobin = 15.5 g/dl
WBC = 7600/mm^3
Neutrophils = 3800/mm^3
Lymphocytes = 3200/mm^3
Monocytes = 200/mm^3
Eosinophils = 300/mm^3
Basophils = 100/mm^3
Platelets = 420 million/mm^3
Morphology = normal

25. Obtain blood from the jugular vein after a 4-hour fast for serum chemistry analysis.

25. The results of the serum chemistry analysis are as follows:
Total protein = 6.0 g/dl
Albumin = 3.5 g/dl

Globulin = 2.5 g/dl
Glucose = 95 mg/dl
BUN = 35 mg/dl
Creatinine = 0.7 mg/dl
Alkaline phosphatase = 52 IU/L
AST = 95 IU/L
ALT = 110 IU/L
Total bilirubin = 0.3 mg/dl

26. Obtain blood from the jugular vein for a feline leukemia virus test.

26. Negative, feline leukemia virus testing is not indicated in ferrets.

27. Swab the ears with an oil coated cotton-tipped applicator and examine the debris under the microscope.

27. Positive for *Otodectes cynotis*.

28. Obtain a blood sample from the jugular vein for the determination of serum estrogen concentration.

28. Normal values for ferrets not established; however, values are within normal dog and cat limits.

29. Collect blood from the jugular vein for measurement of serum thyroxine and triiodothyronine analysis.

29. $T_3 = 0.55$ ng/ml; $T_4 = 1.93$ µg/dl.

30. Administer 0.2 mg dexamethasone intravenously and obtain blood samples at 0, 3, and 5 hours for serum cortisol analysis.

30. 0 hour cortisol = 0.84 µg/dl; 3-hour post-dexamethasone cortisol = 0.17 µg/dl; 5-hour post dexamethasone cortisol = 0.24 µg/dl.

31. Administer 0.5 units ACTH intravenously and obtain blood samples at 0 and 1 hour for serum cortisol analysis.

31. Pre ACTH cortisol = 1.2 ug/dl; 1-hour post-ACTH cortisol = 5.21 µg/dl.

32. Obtain a urine sample for determination of a cortisol:creatinine ratio.

32. Urine cortisol to creatinine ratio = 65:1.

33. Obtain radiographs of the whole body.

33. No abnormal findings.

34. Sedate the ferret and obtain a sample of bone marrow for analysis.

34. Normal.

35. Obtain a blood sample for analysis of blood clotting times.

35. Ferret normal values unknown; within canine and feline normal range.

36. Perform an ultrasonographic examination of the abdomen.

36. No significant findings.

Go to Section D

Section D:

Considering the information you have gained so far, which treatments are most appropriate? (*Choose only those treatments that are relevant to the case at this point.*)

37. Anesthetize the ferret and perform an exploratory laparotomy to look for remnant ovarian tissue.

37. Uterine stump present and normal; no remnant ovarian tissue detectable.

38. Prescribe thyroxine at a dose of 0.01 mg/kg orally every 12 hours and schedule a recheck examination in 2 weeks.

38. No improvement in alopecia; owner seeks second opinion.

39. Prescribe mitotane (o,p'-DDD, Lysodren) at a dose of 50 mg/kg orally once daily for 7 days, then every 72 hours for 8 weeks.

39. No improvement in alopecia.

40. Anesthetize the ferret and perform an ovariohysterectomy.

40. Uterine stump present and normal; no ovarian remnants detected. The alopecia worsens, vulvar swelling continues, and the ferret becomes notably thin.

41. Clean the ears and instill 0.5 mg/kg ivermectin in each ear; repeat in 2 weeks.

41. The crustiness in the ears goes away and the ferret no longer scratches at the ears.

42. No treatment is necessary because the alopecia is seasonal and will resolve within a few months.

42. The alopecia indeed improves within several months; however, it recurs at the same time the following year and the owner seeks a second opinion.

43. Administer 200 IU human chorionic gonado-tropin IM or 20 μg gonadotropin releasing hormone IM; repeat in 2 weeks.

43. No change in the vulvar swelling, but the hair loss worsens.

44. Anesthetize the ferret and perform an exploratory laparotomy.

44. The left adrenal gland is enlarged. Adrenalec-tomy and histopathology reveals an adrenal cortical adenoma. The right adrenal gland and other intraabdominal organs are normal. The vulvar swelling and alopecia resolve within 3 months. Good job!

45. Perform a skin scraping.

45. Negative.

46. Pluck hairs from the periphery of the alopecic areas and place on a dermatophyte test media.

46. No growth.

47. Anesthetize the ferret and perform a skin biopsy for histopathology.

47. Orthokeratotic hyperkeratosis of epidermis and hair follicles, sebaceous gland atrophy; all hair follicles are devoid of hair shafts and in telogen.

48. Prescribe ketoconazole at a dose of 10 mg/kg orally twice daily for 6 weeks.

48. No response to treatment.

END OF PROBLEM

Opening Scene:

A 3½-year-old neutered male ferret is brought to you late one frigid February day at your small animal/exotic pet practice in the midwestern United States. The owner complains that the ferret has been intermittently lethargic and depressed and has been limping on a rear leg. In addition, the ferret has been salivating excessively and pawing at its mouth. These problems seem to be getting progressively worse. Vaccinations, including rabies and canine distemper, are up to date.

Go to Section A

Section A:

What questions would you like to ask the owner? *(Choose only the questions you believe relevant to managing the case at this point.)*

1. What do you normally feed your ferret?

2. How often do you feed your ferret?

3. How often do you bathe your ferret?

4. Is it an indoor or an outdoor ferret?

5. When did you first notice these problems?

6. Have you ever seen your ferret seizure?

7. Does your ferret seem excessively tired after exercise or after sleep?

8. Does your ferret seem to have difficulty eating?

9. Has there been a change in your ferret's water consumption?

10. Has there been any weight loss?

11. Is there any possibility of an injury?

12. Is there a possibility that your ferret ingested a foreign object such as rubber, latex, or plastic?

13. Is the ferret caged when you are not at home or does it have free run of the house?

1. "He eats a high quality ferret food supplemented with Ferritone every other day as a treat."

2. "Food is available free choice."

3. "Once every 2 to 3 weeks."

4. "Indoor exclusively."

5. "For the last few months."

6. "None that I know of."

7. "Yes, he does."

8. "No."

9. "No."

10. "Maybe a little but I'm not really sure."

11. "Someone stepped on his rear foot several weeks ago."

12. "Not that I know of."

13. "It's caged when we're not at home."

Section B:

What physical examination procedures would you perform at this time? *(Choose only those procedures you believe relevant to managing the case at this point.)*

14. Check the skin turgor for evidence of dehydration.

14. No evidence of dehydration.

15. Measure the rectal temperature.

15. 38.5°C.

16. Palpate the peripheral lymph nodes.

16. None feel enlarged.

17. Hold the ferret by its scruff and examine the oral cavity when it opens its mouth.

17. No abnormalities detected. No signs of foreign bodies in the mouth; teeth are in good condition.

18. Check the capillary refill time.

18. Mucous membranes are pink; capillary refill time is less than 2 seconds.

19. Carefully palpate the abdomen while holding the ferret's scruff.

19. Spleen, kidneys, intestines, and bladder all feel normal. No abnormalities or pain responses are noted.

20. Thoroughly palpate all limbs.

20. No abnormal findings.

21. Auscultate the heart and lungs.

21. Normal auscultation.

22. Obtain a body weight on a gram scale.

22. 1.012 kg.

23. Gently compress the anterior thorax.

23. The chest is slightly compressible, within normal limits.

24. Perform a complete neurological examination.

24. No significant abnormalities.

25. Perform a full orthopedic examination of the rear limbs.

25. No significant abnormalities.

Go to Section C

Section C:

What diagnostic/therapeutic procedures would you like to perform? *(Choose only those procedures/therapies that are relevant to managing the case at this point.)*

26. Obtain a stool sample for direct examination and fecal flotation.

26. Negative.

27. Obtain a cardiac ultrasound.

27. Normal.

28. Obtain an ultrasonographic evaluation of the abdomen.

28. Normal with the exception of an enlarged spleen.

29. Obtain blood from the jugular vein for a complete blood count.

29. The complete blood count results show the following:
PCV = 48%
Hemoglobin = 16.5 g/dl
WBC = 5900/mm^3
Neutrophils = 2300/mm^3
Lymphocytes = 3100/mm^3
Monocytes = 100/mm^3
Eosinophils = 100/mm^3
Basophils = 200/mm^3
Platelets = 590 million/mm^3
Morphology = normal

30. Obtain radiographs of the abdomen.

30. No significant findings with the exception of an enlarged spleen.

31. Radiograph the pelvis and hind limbs.

31. No significant findings.

32. Obtain blood from the jugular vein after a 4-hour fast for a serum chemistry analysis.

32. The serum chemistry analysis results show the following:
Total protein = 6.2 g/dl
Albumin = 3.2 g/dl
Globulin = 3.0 g/dl
Glucose = 82 mg/dl
BUN = 21 mg/dl
Creatinine = 0.6 mg/dl
Alkaline phosphatase = 35 IU/L
AST = 110 IU/L
ALT = 95 IU/L
Total bilirubin = 0.3 mg/dl

Go to Section D

Section D:

Considering the information you have gained so far, which treatments are most appropriate? *(Choose only those treatments that are relevant to the case at this point.)*

33. Obtain a sample for cytological examination from the spleen by fine needle aspiration biopsy.

33. No abnormal findings.

34. Obtain a blood sample for a heartworm ELISA test.

34. Normal.

35. Sedate the ferret to perform a bone marrow aspirate for cytological examination.

35. Negative.

36. Obtain a blood sample for a feline leukemia virus test.

36. No significant findings.

37. Perform an ultrasound-guided splenic biopsy.

37. Ferrets are not susceptible to feline leukemia virus.

38. Obtain a blood sample from the jugular vein for a 4- to 6-hour fasting serum glucose and serum insulin concentration.

38. Results:
Glucose = 72 mg/dl
Insulin = 435 pmol/L

39. Administer barium sulfate by stomach tube and perform an upper gastrointestinal radiographic study.

39. No abnormal findings; barium reaches the colon within 3 hours. The owner is dissatisfied with the cost of this diagnostic test.

Go to Section E

Section E:

Considering the information you have gained so far, which treatment is appropriate for this ferret? *(Choose only one.)*

40. Feed high quality protein meals with a dash of Brewer's yeast daily.

40. The ferret initially stabilizes and clinical signs resolve. Gradually the clinical signs return 2 months later. The owner would like a resolution to the problems.

41. Anesthetize the ferret and perform a laparotomy for the purpose of removing the spleen.

41. The ferret's clinical signs worsen and the owner is unhappy.

42. Administer thiacetarsamide at a dose of 2.2 mg/kg intravenously every 12 hours for four treatments.

42. The ferret's clinical signs worsen and the owner is unhappy.

43. Anesthetize the ferret and perform an exploratory laparotomy.

43. Four 1 to 2 mm masses are removed from the pancreas and submitted for histopathology, in addition to liver and pancreatic lymph node biopsies. All other abdominal organs appear normal. Histopathology reveals pancreatic β-cell adenomas or insulinomas. There is no evidence of metastasis to the liver or pancreatic lymph node. Clinical signs recur in 10 months.

44. No treatment necessary.

44. The ferret's clinical signs worsen and the owner is unhappy.

45. Administer lactated Ringer's solution intravenously at a rate of 5 ml/hour constant rate infusion and feline hairball laxative orally; perform a mineral oil enema.

45. The ferret does not improve.

Go to Section F

Section F:

Considering the information you have obtained so far, which additional treatments are appropriate? *(Choose only those responses that you feel appropriate in the management of this case at this point.)*

46. No further treatment is necessary.

46. The ferret's clinical signs worsen and the owner is unhappy.

47. Administer a single dose of ivermectin at a dose of 0.05 mg/kg in 3 to 4 weeks.

47. The ferret's clinical signs worsen and the owner is unhappy.

48. Prescribe pediatric prednisolone syrup at a dose of 0.25 to 1.0 mg/kg/day PO every 12 hours.

48. The ferret's clinical signs improve.

49. Prescribe cyclophosphamide at a dose of 6.25 mg PO every 7 days for three treatments, vincristine at a dose of 0.1 mg IV every 7 days for four treatments, and pediatric prednisolone syrup at a dose of 2 mg/kg PO daily for 5 weeks.

49. The ferret becomes extremely ill and the owner requests a second opinion.

50. Anesthetize the ferret and perform an enterotomy.

50. No abnormalities are detected. The clinical signs worsen.

51. Prescribe ivermectin at a dose of 0.05 mg/kg PO or subcutaneously monthly beginning 1 month before and ending 2 months following the mosquito season.

51. Response noted. Heartworm prophylaxis is recommended in heartworm endemic areas.

52. Prescribe diazoxide at a dose of 10 mg/kg/day PO divided and given every 8 to 12 hours.

52. The clinical signs improve. The dose can be gradually increased to 60 mg/kg/day if needed.

53. Obtain blood samples weekly for the purpose of monitoring complete blood counts.

53. Response noted.

54. Administer amoxicillin at a dose of 10 mg/kg subcutaneously every 12 hours, lactated Ringer's solution intravenously, and feed a liquid diet for 24 hours followed by softened food.

54. The clinical signs continue.

END OF PROBLEM

Opening Scene:

You work in a well-equipped, small animal practice. The owner of a 4-year-old neutered male Sheltie presents the dog to you with a complaint that the dog has difficulty breathing and tires easily. The dog has progressively gotten worse over the past month. The owner notes that the breathing has become more rapid with time. For the past week, the dog has been coughing after minimal exercise such as going up the stairs to the second story of the house. The dog is otherwise fine. He is an indoor dog that has access to a fenced back yard. He lives in the midwestern United States and has not traveled. He is current on his vaccinations, including rabies, and is on monthly heartworm preventative.

Go to Section A

Section A:

What questions would you like to ask the owner? *(Choose only the questions you believe relevant to managing the case at this point.)*

1. Is there any noise associated with his breathing?

    1. "No."

2. Is the cough productive?

    2. "No, he doesn't seem to cough anything up."

3. Does the dog seem to be generally weak?

    3. "No, he's as strong as ever."

4. Is there a possibility of an injury or traumatic incident?

    4. "Not that I know of."

5. Has he had any previous illnesses, injuries, or surgeries?

    5. "No."

6. Does he cough at night or when lying down?

    6. "No."

7. Has he been around any strange or sick dogs?

    7. "No."

8. Has there been a change in the dog's bark?

    8. "No."

9. Has there been any change in your dog's thirst or urination habits?

    9. "No changes."

10. Does your dog appear to favor any leg?

    10. "No."

11. Has your dog collapsed or had any seizures?

    11. "Not that I have seen."

12. Has your dog had any changes in mental attitude or personality?

    12. "His attitude is great."

Section B:

Which physical examination procedures would you perform at this time? *(Choose only the procedures you believe relevant to managing the case at this point.)*

13. Measure the body weight.

14. Measure the rectal body temperature.

15. Take the pulse and heart rate.

16. Measure the respiratory rate and note the character of respirations.

17. Auscultate the lungs.

18. Auscultate the heart.

19. Examine the oral cavity.

20. Palpate the peripheral lymph nodes.

21. Palpate the abdomen.

22. Examine the skin.

23. Examine the ears, eyes, and nose.

24. Check for a jugular pulse.

25. Assess cranial nerves, mental status, postural and spinal reflexes, gait and proprioception.

26. Palpate the muscles and bones, and flex and extend the joints.

13. 12 kg.

14. 38.3°C.

15. The heart rate is 108 beats per minute; the pulse is strong and regular.

16. The respiration rate is 72 per minute and shallow.

17. Lung sounds are absent ventrally and harsh dorsally.

18. Heart sounds are muffled but normal.

19. Normal; mucous membranes are pink; capillary refill time is 1 second.

20. Normal.

21. Normal.

22. Normal.

23. No abnormalities.

24. Jugular pulses are not present.

25. The dog is neurologically normal.

26. The musculoskeletal system is normal.

Go to Section C

Section C:

Which diagnostic procedures would you perform? *(Choose only the procedures you believe relevant to managing the case at this point.)*

27. Collect blood for a complete blood count.

27. The complete blood count results show the following:
PCV = 42%
Hb = 15.2 g/dl
RBC = 7.5 million/mm^3
MCV = 62 fl
MCHC = 32 g/dl

MCH = 23 pg
WBC = 11,800/mm^3
Segs = 9800/mm^3
Bands = 0/mm^3
Lymphocytes = 1200/mm^3
Monocytes = 600/mm^3
Eosinophils = 200/mm^3
Basophils = 0/mm^3
Platelets = 245,000/mm^3
Total protein = 6.5 g/dl

28. Collect blood for a serum chemistry profile.

28. The serum chemistry profile results show the following:
Glucose = 105 mg/dl
BUN = 16 mg/dl
Creatinine = 1.0 mg/dl
Albumin = 3.5 g/dl
Total protein = 6.5 g/dl
ALT = 60 IU/L
GGT = 1 IU/L
SAP = 65 IU/L
Amylase = 250 IU/L
Cholesterol = 100 mg/dl
Sodium = 145 mEq/L
Potassium = 4.4 mEq/L
Chloride = 112 mEq/L
Calcium = 9.6 mg/dl
Phosphorus = 3.6 mg/dl
Total bilirubin = 0.1 mg/dl
Total CO$_2$ = 20 mmol/L

29. Collect urine for a urinalysis.

29. The urine was collected by cystocentesis.
Color = yellow
Character = clear
Specific gravity= 1.038
pH = 6.5
Protein = negative
Glucose = negative
Ketones = negative
Bilirubin = 1+
Urobilinogen = negative
Blood = negative
WBC = 1-3/hpf
RBC = 3-5/hpf
Epithelial cells/hpf = occasionally
Bacteria = negative
Casts = negative
Crystals = 1+struvite
Sperm = negative
Fat = negative

30. Collect blood to perform a Coomb's test.

30. Negative.

31. Exercise the dog and perform a Tensilon test.

31. The dog did not collapse when exercising so the test could not be performed.

32. Collect blood for a serum antiacetylcholine receptor antibody titer.

32. The serum antiacetylcholine receptor antibody titer result is 1:2.

33. Collect blood for a *Borrelia* titer.

33. The *Borrelia* titer result is 1:4.

34. Collect blood for an *Ehrlichia canis* titer.

34. The *Ehrlichia canis* titer result is 1:2.

35. Collect blood for heartworm serology.

35. Negative.

36. Collect blood for serial blood glucose measurement.

36. The serial blood glucose measurement results are 100 mg/dl, 98 mg/dl, 96 mg/dl, and 102 mg/dl.

37. Perform an electrocardiogram.

37. Normal sinus rhythm.

38. Perform an echocardiogram.

38. Normal cardiac structure and function.

39. Obtain chest radiographs.

39. Soft tissue density in the ventral thorax silhouetting the heart; consistent with a large amount of pleural fluid.

40. Obtain abdominal radiographs.

40. Normal.

41. Perform fluoroscopy of the trachea.

41. Normal trachea.

42. Perform an abdominocentesis to collect abdominal fluid.

42. No fluid obtained.

43. Collect blood for aerobic and anaerobic blood cultures.

43. No growth.

44. Perform a thoracocentesis to collect thoracic fluid.

44. 750 ml of pink, milky fluid removed.

Go to Section D

Section D:

Considering the information you have gained so far, what further diagnostic tests would you like to perform? (*Choose only the tests you believe relevant to managing the case at this point.*)

45. Perform a 24-hour electrocardiogram.

45. Normal sinus rhythm.

46. Perform abdominal exploratory surgery.

46. No abnormal findings.

47. Perform a thoracic ultrasound.

47. Moderate amount of pleural effusion; no masses identified.

48. Obtain respiratory samples by transtracheal wash or bronchoalveolar lavage.

48. Normal respiratory epithelial cells with low numbers of macrophages; no organisms seen.

49. Collect blood for serum titers for *Blastomyces, Histoplasma,* and *Coccidioidomyces.*

49. Negative.

50. Collect blood for an antinuclear antibody or *Lupus erythematosus* test.

50. Negative.

51. Examine the thoracic fluid microscopically.

51. 75% small lymphocytes, 20% mesothelial cells, 5% neutrophils; no organisms seen.

52. Collect respiratory samples by transthoracic aspirate.

52. Normal respiratory epithelial cells and peripheral blood.

53. Collect blood and thoracic fluid for triglyceride and cholesterol determinations.

53.

	Serum	Fluid
Triglyceride	60 mg/dl	520 mg/dl
Cholesterol	100 mg/dl	80 mg/dl

54. Perform cardiac catheterization and angiography.

54. Normal cardiac structure and function.

55. Obtain radiographs of joints.

55. Normal joints.

56. Perform an arthrocentesis.

56. WBC = 300/mm^3; predominately mononuclear with rare synovial cells.

Go to Section E

Section E:

Which course of action would you take? *(Choose only one.)*

57. Prescribe prednisone at immunosuppressive dosages to be tapered over the next 3 months to alternate day therapy.

57. End of problem.

58. Prescribe digoxin, enalopril, and furosemide and give the owner a guarded prognosis.

58. End of problem.

59. Prescribe theophylline and an antiinflammatory dose of prednisone to be tapered over the next month to alternate day therapy.

59. End of problem.

60. Place the dog on a low fat diet and medium chain triglyceride oil and reassess in 1 week.

60. End of problem.

61. Place the dog on a schedule of frequent feedings of canned dog food with corn syrup added and prescribe diazoxide and a low dose of prednisone daily.

61. End of problem.

62. Prescribe a 3-week course of doxycycline and reevaluate the dog then.

62. End of problem.

END OF PROBLEM

Opening Scene:

The owner of a 3-year-old neutered male domestic shorthaired cat presents her cat to you with a problem of nasal discharge and sneezing of 6 weeks duration. The problem began with a clear nasal discharge and episodes of sneezing 6 weeks earlier. Gradually, the nasal discharge has become green and thick with occasional flecks of blood in it. The cat's appetite is slightly depressed but he has not lost an appreciable amount of weight. The cat goes outdoors during the day but usually sleeps indoors at night. He is current on his vaccinations, including rabies.

Go to Section A

Section A:

What questions would you like to ask the owner? (*Choose only the questions you believe relevant to managing the case at this point.*)

1. Is there any noise associated with his breathing?

    1. "Yes, he rattles and snorts."

2. Is the nasal discharge unilateral or bilateral?

    2. "It is primarily from the right side."

3. Do you have other animals?

    3. "No, he's our only pet."

4. Is there a possibility of an injury or traumatic incident?

    4. "Not that I know of."

5. Has he had any previous illnesses, injuries, or surgeries?

    5. "No."

6. How frequently does he sneeze?

    6. "It seems like 5 to 10 episodes a day, at least."

7. Has there been any ocular discharge?

    7. "No."

8. Have you noticed anything that triggers him to sneeze?

    8. "He sneezes the most after he gets up in the morning."

9. Has there been any change in your cat's thirst or urination habits?

    9. "No changes."

10. Does your cat appear to be lame?

    10. "No."

11. Has your cat collapsed or had any seizures?

    11. "Not that I have seen."

12. Has your cat had any changes in mental attitude or personality?

    12. "His attitude is great."

13. Has your cat been vomiting or had any diarrhea?

    13. "No."

Go to Section B

Section B:

Which physical examination procedures would you perform at this time? *(Choose only the procedures you believe relevant to managing the case at this point.)*

14. Measure the body weight.

14. 4.6 kg.

15. Measure the rectal body temperature.

15. 38.3°C.

16. Take the pulse and heart rate.

16. The heart rate is 144 beats per minute; the pulse is strong and regular.

17. Measure the respiratory rate and note the character of respirations.

17. The respiratory rate is 16 per minute. An inspiratory stridor is noted.

18. Auscultate the lungs.

18. Lung sounds are normal.

19. Auscultate the heart.

19. Heart sounds are normal.

20. Examine the oral cavity.

20. Mild dental tartar; mucous membranes are pink; capillary refill time is 1 second.

21. Palpate the peripheral lymph nodes.

21. Normal.

22. Palpate the abdomen.

22. Normal.

23. Examine the skin.

23. Normal.

24. Examine the ears, eyes, and nose.

24. No abnormalities with the ears and eyes; right-sided mucopurulent nasal discharge present.

25. Check for air movement through both nostrils.

25. No air movement through right nostril.

26. Assess cranial nerves, mental status, postural and spinal reflexes, gait and proprioception.

26. The cat is neurologically normal.

27. Palpate the muscles and bones, and flex and extend the joints.

27. The musculoskeletal system is normal.

28. Perform a funduscopic examination.

28. The funduscopic exam is normal.

Go to Section C

Section C:

Which diagnostic procedures would you perform? *(Choose only the procedures you believe relevant to managing the case at this point.)*

29. Collect blood for a complete blood count.

29. The complete blood count results show the following:
PCV = 42%
Hb = 18.2 g/dl

RBC = 11.5 million/mm^3
MCV = 42 fl
MCHC = 33 g/dl
MCH = 15 pg
WBC = 14,800/mm^3
Segs = 11,800/mm^3
Bands = 0/mm^3
Lymphocytes = 1200/mm^3
Monocytes = 1600/mm^3
Eosinophils = 200/mm^3
Basophils = 0/mm^3
Platelets = 245,000/mm^3
Total protein = 8.5 g/dl

30. Collect blood for a serum chemistry profile.

30. The serum chemistry profile results show the following:
Glucose = 105 mg/dl
BUN = 16 mg/dl
Creatinine = 1.0 mg/dl
Albumin = 3.5 g/dl
Total protein = 8.5 g/dl
ALT = 60 IU/L
GGT = 1 IU/L
SAP = 65 IU/L
Amylase = 250 IU/L
Cholesterol = 100 mg/dl
Sodium = 145 mEq/L
Potassium = 4.4 mEq/L
Chloride = 112 mEq/L
Calcium = 9.6 mg/dl
Phosphorus = 3.6 mg/dl
Total bilirubin = 0.1 mg/dl
Total CO$_2$ = 20 mmol/L

31. Collect urine for a urinalysis.

31. The urine was collected by cystocentesis.
Color = yellow
Character = clear
Specific gravity = 1.058
pH = 6.5
Protein = negative
Glucose = negative
Ketones = negative
Bilirubin = negative
Urobilinogen = negative
Blood = negative
WBC = 1-3/hpf
RBC = 3-5/hpf
Epithelial cells/hpf = occasionally
Bacteria = negative
Casts = negative
Crystals = 1+struvite
Sperm = negative
Fat = negative

32. Collect blood for a feline leukemia virus test.

32. Negative.

33. Collect blood for a feline immunodeficiency virus test.

33. Negative.

34. Collect blood for a coagulation profile.

34. Normal.

35. Collect a sample of nasal discharge and examine microscopically.

35. Degenerate neutrophils with numerous intracellular cocci and rods.

36. Perform a conjunctival scraping and examine microscopically.

36. Normal conjunctival epithelial cells.

37. Collect a sample of nasal discharge for aerobic culture and antibiotic sensitivity.

37. Light growth of *Staphylococcus aureus, Streptococcus* spp, and *E. coli;* sensitive to all antibiotics.

38. Collect lower respiratory samples by transtracheal wash.

38. Normal respiratory epithelial cells, occasional macrophages; no organisms seen.

39. Perform an electrocardiogram.

39. Normal sinus rhythm.

40. Refer the cat to a specialist for an echocardiogram.

40. Normal cardiac structure and function.

41. Obtain chest radiographs.

41. Normal.

42. Obtain abdominal radiographs.

42. Normal.

43. Perform fluoroscopy of the trachea.

43. Normal trachea.

44. Perform an abdominocentesis for collection of abdominal fluid.

44. No fluid obtained.

45. Collect blood for aerobic and anaerobic cultures.

45. No growth.

46. Perform a thoracocentesis for collection of thoracic fluid.

46. No fluid obtained.

Go to Section D

Section D:

Considering the information you have gained so far, what further diagnostic tests would you like to perform? (*Choose only the tests you believe relevant to managing the case at this point.*)

47. Anesthetize the cat for skull radiographs.

47. Soft tissue density filling right nasal cavity; no bone lysis.

48. Perform exploratory surgery of the nasal passages and sinuses.

48. No evidence of neoplasia or foreign objects; biopsies are pending.

49. Anesthetize the cat for rhinoscopy.

49. Mucopurulent nasal discharge obscures view of nasal passage; no obvious masses or foreign objects.

50. Collect lower respiratory samples by bronchoalveolar lavage.

50. Normal respiratory epithelial cells with low numbers of macrophages; no organisms seen.

51. Collect blood for *Herpes* serology.

51. The result of the *Herpes* serology is 1:4.

52. Collect blood for *Cryptococcus* serology.

52. The result of the *Cryptococcus* serology is 1:256.

53. Collect blood for feline infectious peritonitis virus serology.

53. The result of the feline infectious peritonitis virus serology is 1:100.

54. Perform a transthoracic aspirate.

54. Normal respiratory epithelial cells and peripheral blood.

55. Collect blood for *Toxoplasma* serology.

55. The result of the *Toxoplasma* serology is IgG = 1:32 and IgM = 1:16.

56. Collect aqueous humor by aqueocentesis.

56. Normal.

57. Anesthetize the cat and collect cerebrospinal fluid.

57. 0 cells; protein = 5 mg/dl; pandy is negative.

Go to Section E

Section E:

Which course of action would you take? *(Choose only one.)*

58. Prescribe prednisone at immunosuppressive dosages to be tapered over the next 3 months to alternate day therapy.

58. End of problem.

59. Pull the right upper canine tooth and prescribe amoxicillin for 2 weeks.

59. End of problem.

60. Prescribe theophylline, chlorpheniramine, and an antiinflammatory dose of prednisone to be tapered over the next month to alternate day therapy.

60. End of problem.

61. Treat the cat with ivermectin weekly for four treatments.

61. End of problem.

62. Refer the cat for radiation therapy.

62. End of problem.

63. Prescribe a 3-week course of clindamycin and reevaluate the cat at the end of that time.

63. End of problem.

64. Prescribe ketoconazole and reevaluate the cat in 1 week.

64. End of problem.

END OF PROBLEM

Opening Scene:

The owners of a 12-year-old spayed female miniature poodle present her to you at your predominately small animal practice with a history of a cough of 3 days duration. The cough occurs episodically, mostly at night. The dog is otherwise normal. She has a good appetite and has had no vomiting or diarrhea. She seems to drink a normal amount of water and urinates normally. She had all her vaccinations, including rabies, 3 months ago. She is primarily an indoor dog and has access to a fenced-in backyard. The location is the midwestern United States.

Go to Section A

Section A:

What questions would you like to ask the owner? *(Choose only the questions you believe relevant to managing the case at this point.)*

1. Has there been any exercise intolerance?	1. "Not really, but she has slowed down over the last 2 years."
2. Is the cough productive?	2. "No, she doesn't seem to cough anything up."
3. Does she cough when excited?	3. "No."
4. Is there a possibility of an injury or traumatic incident?	4. "Not that I know of."
5. Has she had any previous illnesses, injuries, or surgeries?	5. "Only her spay at 6 months of age."
6. Is she on heartworm preventative?	6. "No."
7. Has she been around any strange or sick dogs?	7. "No."
8. Does your dog have any nasal or ocular discharge?	8. "Just a drop of clear fluid now and then."
9. Has there been a change in the dog's bark?	9. "No changes."
10. Does the dog seem to be generally weak?	10. "No."
11. Does your dog appear to favor any leg?	11. "No."
12. Has your dog collapsed or had any seizures?	12. "Not that I have seen."
13. Has your dog had any changes in mental attitude or personality?	13. "Her attitude is great."
14. Do you normally use a collar or harness with your dog?	14. "We use a collar but she's rarely on a leash."

Section B:

Which physical examination procedures would you perform at this time? *(Choose only the procedures you believe relevant to managing the case at this point.)*

15. Measure the body weight.

16. Measure the rectal body temperature.

17. Take the pulse and heart rate.

18. Measure the respiratory rate and note the character of respirations.

19. Auscultate the lungs.

20. Auscultate the heart.

21. Examine the oral cavity.

22. Palpate the trachea.

23. Palpate the peripheral lymph nodes.

24. Palpate the abdomen.

25. Examine the skin.

26. Examine the ears, eyes, and nose.

27. Check for a jugular pulse.

28. Assess cranial nerves, mental status, postural and spinal reflexes, gait and proprioception.

29. Palpate the muscles and bones, and flex and extend the joints.

15. 14 kg.

16. 38.3°C.

17. The heart rate is 120 beats per minute; the pulse is strong and regular.

18. The respiratory rate is 20 per minute and normal.

19. Lung sounds are harsh.

20. There is a grade III/VI holosystolic murmur that is loudest over the left apex.

21. The oral cavity is normal; mucous membranes are pink; capillary refill time is 1 second.

22. The trachea palpates normally and no cough can be elicited.

23. Normal.

24. Normal.

25. Normal.

26. No abnormalities.

27. Jugular pulses are not present.

28. The dog is neurologically normal.

29. The musculoskeletal system is normal.

Go to Section C

Section C:

Which diagnostic procedures would you perform? *(Choose only the procedures you believe relevant to managing the case at this point.)*

30. Collect blood for a complete blood count.

30. The complete blood count results show the following:
PCV = 42%
Hb = 15.2 g/dl

RBC = 7.5 million/mm³
MCV = 62 fl
MCHC = 32 g/dl
MCH = 23 pg
WBC = 11,800/mm³
Segs = 9800/mm³
Bands = 0/mm³
Lymphocytes = 1200/mm³
Monocytes = 600/mm³
Eosinophils = 200/mm³
Basophils = 0/mm³
Platelets = 245,000/mm³
Total protein = 6.5 g/dl

31. Collect blood for a serum chemistry profile.

31. The serum chemistry profile results show the following:
Glucose = 105 mg/dl
BUN = 16 mg/dl
Creatinine = 1.0 mg/dl
Albumin = 3.5 g/dl
Total protein = 6.5 g/dl
ALT = 60 IU/L
GGT = 1 IU/L
SAP = 365 IU/L
Amylase = 250 IU/L
Cholesterol = 100 mg/dl
Sodium = 145 mEq/L
Potassium = 4.4 mEq/L
Chloride = 112 mEq/L
Calcium = 9.6 mg/dl
Phosphorus = 3.6 mg/dl
Total bilirubin = 0.1 mg/dl
Total CO_2 = 20 mmol/L

32. Collect urine for a urinalysis.

32. The urine was collected by cystocentesis.
Color = yellow
Character = clear
Specific gravity = 1.038
pH = 6.5
Protein = negative
Glucose = negative
Ketones = negative
Bilirubin = negative
Urobilinogen = negative
Blood = negative
WBC = 1-3/hpf
RBC = 3-5/hpf
Epithelial cells/hpf = occasional
Bacteria = negative
Casts = negative
Crystals = 1+struvite
Sperm = negative
Fat = negative

33. Collect blood for a Knott's test.

33. Negative.

34. Anesthetize the dog for skull radiographs.

34. Normal.

35. Perform a laryngeal examination under sedation.

35. Normal.

36. Refer the dog to a specialist for rhinoscopy.

36. Normal.

37. Refer the dog to a specialist for bronchoscopy.

37. Normal.

38. Obtain chest radiographs.

38. The thoracic wall is normal; no pleural space disease is noted; the lung fields have mild interstitial changes compatible with age; examination of the pulmonary vessels reveals mild dilation of the veins; moderate left atrial enlargement.

39. Obtain abdominal radiographs.

39. Normal.

40. Perform an electrocardiogram.

40. Normal sinus rhythm; occasional premature atrial contractions.

41. Obtain feces for fecal flotation.

41. Negative.

42. Obtain feces for fecal sedimentation.

42. Negative.

43. Perform fluoroscopy of the trachea.

43. Normal.

44. Collect blood for fasting and postprandial bile acid determination.

44. Preprandial = 5 μmol/L; postprandial = 10 μmol/L.

45. Collect blood for aerobic and anaerobic cultures.

45. No growth.

46. Collect thoracic fluid by thoracocentesis.

46. No fluid obtained.

Go to Section D

Section D:

Considering the information you have gained so far, what further diagnostic tests would you like to perform? *(Choose only the tests you believe relevant to managing the case at this point.)*

47. Perform a 24-hour electrocardiogram.

47. Normal.

48. Collect lower respiratory samples by trans-tracheal wash.

48. Normal respiratory epithelial cells with low numbers of macrophages; no organisms seen.

49. Refer the dog to a specialist for collection of lower respiratory samples by bronchoalveolar lavage.

49. 75% macrophages, 20% normal respiratory epithelial cells; 5% healthy neutrophils.

50. Collect lower respiratory samples by trans-thoracic aspirate.

50. Normal respiratory epithelial cells and peripheral blood.

51. Collect blood for serum titers for *Blastomyces, Histoplasma,* and *Coccidioidomyces.*

51. Negative.

52. Collect blood for heartworm serology.

52. Negative.

53. Refer the dog to a specialist for an echocardiogram.

53. Left atrial enlargement with moderate to severe mitral valve insufficiency; normal cardiac function.

54. Anesthetize the dog and perform exploratory surgery of the thorax.

54. Mild cardiomegaly with no other abnormalities.

55. Ultrasound the abdomen.

55. Normal abdominal structures.

56. Refer the dog to a specialist for cardiac catheterization and angiography.

56. Mitral regurgitation and left atrial enlargement.

Go to Section E

Section E:

Which course of action would you take? (*Choose only one.*)

57. Prescribe prednisone at immunosuppressive dosages to be tapered over the next 3 months to alternate day therapy.

57. End of problem.

58. Prescribe digoxin and furosemide and give the owner a guarded prognosis.

58. End of problem.

59. Prescribe theophylline and an antiinflammatory dose of prednisone to be tapered over the next month to alternate day therapy.

59. End of problem.

60. Prescribe fenbendazole for 3 days and schedule a recheck examination in 1 month.

60. End of problem.

61. Prescribe a low-salt diet, enalopril, and furosemide and recheck in 2 weeks.

61. End of problem.

62. Prescribe a 3-week course of doxycycline and reevaluate the dog at the end of that time.

62. End of problem.

END OF PROBLEM

Opening Scene:

The owner of a 5-year-old neutered male domestic shorthaired cat presents her cat to you with acute paralysis of his back legs. He was fine earlier in the day, but about 1 hour ago he yowled in pain and began dragging his back legs behind him. He is an indoor and outdoor cat. He is current on his vaccinations, including rabies.

Go to Section A

Section A:

What questions would you like to ask the owner? (*Choose only the questions you believe relevant to managing the case at this point.*)

1. Is there any possibility of injury or traumatic incident?

2. Has he ever had this problem before?

3. Do you have other animals?

4. Is he on any medications?

5. Has he had any previous illnesses, injuries, or surgeries?

6. Has he exhibited any difficulty breathing?

7. Has there been any ocular or nasal discharge?

8. Has he seemed less playful or less active in the recent past?

9. Has there been any change in your cat's thirst or urination habits?

10. Has your cat vomited or had diarrhea recently?

11. Has your cat collapsed or had any seizures?

12. Has your cat had any changes in mental attitude or personality?

13. When was your cat vaccinated last?

1. "It's very unlikely."

2. "No."

3. "No, he's our only pet."

4. "No."

5. "No. Just his neuter surgery."

6. "Today in the car, he was panting."

7. "No."

8. "Not that I know of."

9. "No changes."

10. "No."

11. "Not that I have seen."

12. "No."

13. "Three months ago."

Section B:

Which physical examination procedures would you perform at this time? (*Choose only the procedures you believe relevant to managing the case at this point.*)

14. Measure the body weight.

14. 3.6 kg.

15. Measure the rectal body temperature.

15. 38.3°C.

16. Take the pulse and heart rate.

16. The heart rate is 240 beats per minute; the pulse is not detectable.

17. Measure the respiratory rate and note the character of respirations.

17. The respiratory rate is 16 per minute.

18. Auscultate the lungs.

18. Lung sounds are normal.

19. Auscultate the heart.

19. Grade III/VI systolic murmur; point of maximal intensity is right base.

20. Examine the oral cavity.

20. Mild dental tartar; mucous membranes are pale pink; capillary refill time is 3 seconds.

21. Palpate the peripheral lymph nodes.

21. Normal.

22. Palpate the abdomen.

22. Normal.

23. Examine the skin.

23. Normal.

24. Examine the ears, eyes, and nose.

24. No abnormalities.

25. Examine the nail beds.

25. Nail beds of rear legs are purple in color.

26. Assess cranial nerves, mental status, postural and spinal reflexes, gait and proprioception.

26. Cranial nerves and front legs are normal; absent proprioception and depressed reflexes bilaterally in rear limbs.

27. Palpate the muscles and bones, and flex and extend the joints.

27. The musculoskeletal system is normal with the exception of the rear legs; palpation of all muscle groups in rear legs elicits a strong pain response.

28. Perform a funduscopic examination.

28. The funduscopic exam is normal.

Section C:

Which diagnostic procedures would you perform? *(Choose only the procedures you believe relevant to managing the case at this point.)*

29. Collect blood for a complete blood count.

29. The complete blood count results show the following:
PCV = 42%
Hb = 18.2 g/dl
RBC = 11.5 million/mm^3
MCV = 42 fl
MCHC = 33 g/dl
MCH = 15 pg
WBC = 14,800/mm^3
Segs = 11,800/mm^3
Bands = 0/mm^3
Lymphocytes = 1200/mm^3
Monocytes = 1600/mm^3
Eosinophils = 200/mm^3
Basophils = 0/mm^3
Platelets = 245,000/mm^3
Total protein = 8.5 g/dl

30. Collect blood for a serum chemistry profile.

30. The serum chemistry profile results show the following:
Glucose = 165 mg/dl
BUN = 16 mg/dl
Creatinine = 1.0 mg/dl
Albumin = 3.5 g/dl
Total protein = 8.5 g/dl
ALT = 60 IU/L
GGT = 1 IU/L
SAP = 65 IU/L
Amylase = 250 IU/L
Cholesterol = 100 mg/dl
Sodium = 145 mEq/L
Potassium = 4.4 mEq/L
Chloride = 112 mEq/L
Calcium = 9.6 mg/dl
Phosphorous = 3.6 mg/dl
Total bilirubin = 0.1 mg/dl
Total CO2 = 20 mmol/L

31. Collect urine for a urinalysis.

31. The urine was collected by cystocentesis.
Color = yellow
Character = clear
Specific gravity = 1.058
pH = 6.5
Protein = negative
Glucose = negative
Ketones = negative
Bilirubin = negative
Urobilinogen = negative
Blood = negative

WBC = 1-3/hpf
RBC = 3-5/hpf
Epithelial cells/hpf = occasionally
Bacteria = negative
Casts = negative
Crystals = 1+struvite
Sperm = negative
Fat = negative

32. Collect blood for a feline leukemia virus test.

32. Negative.

33. Collect blood for a feline immunodeficiency virus test.

33. Negative.

34. Collect blood for a coagulation profile.

34. Normal.

35. Clip a toenail past the quick.

35. Nail does not bleed when clipped at the quick.

36. Obtain survey spinal radiographs (awake).

36. Normal.

37. Obtain chest radiographs.

37. Biatrial heart enlargement.

38. Obtain abdominal radiographs.

38. Normal.

39. Perform an electrocardiogram.

39. Normal sinus rhythm; tall R waves.

40. Collect blood for AST and creatine kinase determination.

40. AST = 10,000 IU/L; CK = 12,500 IU/L.

Go to Section D

Section D:

Considering the information you have gained so far, what further diagnostic tests would you like to perform? (*Choose only the tests you believe relevant to managing the case at this point.*)

41. Anesthetize the cat and perform spinal radiographs and a myelogram.

41. Normal.

42. Obtain an echocardiogram.

42. Hypertrophic cardiomyopathy.

43. Anesthetize the cat and perform a muscle biopsy.

43. Results pending.

44. Anesthetize the cat for electromyography.

44. Results pending.

45. Collect blood for feline infectious peritonitis virus serology.

45. Negative.

46. Collect blood for *Toxoplasma* serology.

46. IgG = 1:32, IgM = 1:16.

47. Collect aqueous humor by aqueocentesis.

47. Normal.

48. Anesthetize the cat and collect cerebrospinal fluid.

48. Normal.

49. Collect blood for thyroid hormone analysis.

49. $T_4 = 2.5$ μg/dl.

Go to Section E

Section E:

Which course of action would you take? *(Choose only one.)*

50. Prescribe prednisone at antiinflammatory dosages to be tapered over the next 3 weeks to alternate day therapy.

50. End of problem.

51. Perform a hemilaminectomy at L2-3.

51. End of problem.

52. Prescribe high dose clindamycin for 21 days.

52. End of problem.

53. Prescribe diltiazem, aspirin, and give supportive care.

53. End of problem.

54. Refer the cat to a specialist for radiation therapy.

54. End of problem.

55. Prescribe immunosuppressive doses of prednisone to be tapered over the next 3 months to alternate day therapy.

55. End of problem.

END OF PROBLEM

Opening Scene:

The owners of a 12-year-old spayed female Miniature schnauzer present her to you at your urban small animal practice with a history of vomiting of 1 day duration. The dog has vomited approximately 15 to 20 times since yesterday. She also has not eaten since the day before yesterday. She had all her vaccinations, including rabies, 3 months ago. She is primarily an indoor dog and has access to a fenced-in backyard.

Go to Section A

Section A:

What questions would you like to ask the owner? (*Choose only the questions you believe relevant to managing the case at this point.*)

1. What does the vomitus look like?

1. "The vomitus is a yellowish foam, and the last few times she has vomited it has had flecks of blood in it."

2. Did she get into the garbage or was she fed table scraps before getting sick?

2. "She can't get in the garbage but we do give her table scraps occasionally. Two days ago, she was given some skin from the chicken we cooked."

3. Is there any possibility of exposure to toxins, such as insecticides or antifreeze?

3. "No."

4. Has she had similar problems before this episode?

4. "Not that I know of."

5. Has she had any previous illnesses, injuries, or surgeries?

5. "Only her spay at 6 months of age."

6. Is she receiving any medications?

6. "No."

7. Has she been around any strange or sick dogs?

7. "No."

8. What is the character of the stool?

8. "It is dark brown and watery."

9. How frequently is she having a bowel movement?

9. "She goes three to four times a day."

10. Is there any blood or mucus in the stool?

10. "No."

11. Has your dog been coughing?

11. "No."

12. Has your dog collapsed or had any seizures?

12. "Not that I have seen."

13. Has your dog had any changes in mental attitude or personality?

13. "She is not like herself at all. She just lays around and is not interested in anything."

14. Has there been any change in your dog's water consumption or urinary habits?

14. "She tries to drink but then vomits it up. She seems to be urinating less than normal."

Section B:

Which physical examination procedures would you perform at this time? (*Choose only the procedures you believe relevant to managing the case at this point.*)

15. Measure the body weight.

15. 10 kg.

16. Measure the rectal body temperature.

16. 40.0°C.

17. Take the pulse and heart rate.

17. The heart rate is 180 beats per minute; the pulse is strong and regular.

18. Measure the respiratory rate and note the character of respirations.

18. The respiratory rate is 36 per minute and normal.

19. Auscultate the lungs.

19. Lung sounds are normal.

20. Auscultate the heart.

20. Heart sounds are normal.

21. Examine the oral cavity.

21. The oral cavity is normal; mucous membranes are pink; capillary refill time is 2.5 seconds.

22. Assess the hydration status.

22. Skin turgor is significantly reduced and the mucous membranes are dry and tacky.

23. Palpate the peripheral lymph nodes.

23. Normal.

24. Palpate the abdomen.

24. Abdominal pain is evident, especially in the cranial abdomen. No free abdominal fluid is detected, nor are any masses identified.

25. Examine the skin.

25. Normal.

26. Examine the ears, eyes, and nose.

26. No abnormalities.

27. Check for a jugular pulse.

27. Jugular pulses are not present.

28. Assess cranial nerves, mental status, postural and spinal reflexes, gait and proprioception.

28. The dog is neurologically normal.

29. Palpate the muscles and bones, and flex and extend the joints.

29. The musculoskeletal system is normal.

Section C:

Which diagnostic procedures would you perform? *(Choose only the procedures you believe relevant to managing the case at this point.)*

30. Collect blood for a complete blood count.

30. The complete blood count results show the following:
PCV = 42%
Hb = 15.2 g/dl
RBC = 7.5 million/mm^3
MCV = 62 fl
MCHC = 32 g/dl
MCH = 23 pg
WBC = 31,800/mm^3
Segs = 27,600/mm^3
Bands = 1200/mm^3
Lymphocytes = 1000/mm^3
Monocytes = 2000/mm^3
Eosinophils = 0/mm^3
Basophils = 0/mm^3
Platelets = 245,000/mm^3
Total protein = 7.5 g/dl

31. Collect blood for a serum chemistry profile.

31. The serum chemistry profile sample is lipemic.
Glucose = 165 mg/dl
BUN = 86 mg/dl
Creatinine = 6.0 mg/dl
Albumin = 4.5 g/dl
Total protein = 6.5 g/dl
ALT = 360 IU/L
GGT = 6 IU/L
SAP = 365 IU/L
Cholesterol = 400 mg/dl
Sodium = 134 mEq/L
Potassium = 2.4 mEq/L
Chloride = 92 mEq/L
Calcium = 7.6 mg/dl
Phosphorus = 7.6 mg/dl
Total bilirubin = 0.1 mg/dl
Total CO_2 = 10 mmol/L

32. Collect urine for a urinalysis.

32. The urine was collected by cystocentesis.
Color = yellow
Character = clear
Specific gravity = 1.048
pH = 6.0
Protein = negative
Glucose = negative
Ketones = negative
Bilirubin = 3+
Urobilinogen = trace
Blood = negative
WBC = 1-3/hpf
RBC = 3-5/hpf

Epithelial cells/hpf = occasionally
Bacteria = negative
Casts = negative
Crystals = negative
Sperm = negative
Fat = negative

33. Collect blood for a Knott's test.

33. Negative.

34. Collect blood for amylase and lipase determination.

34. Amylase 1650 IU/L; Lipase 500 IU/L.

35. Collect blood pre- and post-ACTH administration for determination of serum cortisol concentrations.

35. Pre-ACTH cortisol = 6.6 µg/dl; post-ACTH cortisol = 14 µg/dl.

36. Perform abdominal paracentesis for collection of abdominal fluid.

36. A few drops of serosanguinous fluid are obtained; cytology is consistent with a suppurative, nonseptic peritonitis.

37. Collect vomitus and blood for toxicologic screening.

37. No toxins identified.

38. Obtain chest radiographs.

38. Normal.

39. Obtain abdominal radiographs.

39. There is a mild amount of gas in the descending duodenum. Detail is poor in the right anterior quadrant of the abdomen. No masses or foreign bodies are identified. The liver and kidneys appear normal in size and shape.

40. Perform an electrocardiogram.

40. Sinus tachycardia.

41. Obtain feces for fecal flotation.

41. Negative.

42. Obtain feces for fecal cytology.

42. Normal.

43. Pass a urinary catheter to assess patency of the urethra.

43. The catheter passes into the bladder without resistance; 100 ml of urine is removed.

44. Collect blood for thyroid hormone determination.

44. $T_4 = 1.0$ µg/dl.

45. Collect blood for aerobic and anaerobic bacterial cultures.

45. No growth.

46. Perform an intravenous glucose tolerance test.

46.

Time (minutes)	Blood Glucose (mg/dl)
0	165
15	260
30	325
60	304
90	295

Section D:

Considering the information you have gained so far, what further diagnostic tests would you like to perform? *(Choose only the tests you believe relevant to managing the case at this point.)*

47. Collect blood for serum triglyceride determination.

47. Serum triglycerides = 235 mg/dl.

48. Collect blood for ethylene glycol testing.

48. Negative.

49. Perform a barium upper gastrointestinal series.

49. Normal.

50. Perform an endogenous creatinine clearance.

50. 2.9 mg/kg/min.

51. Perform a water deprivation test.

51. Scheduled.

52. Anesthetize the dog and perform upper gastrointestinal endoscopy.

52. No gross abnormalities noted; biopsies are pending.

53. Collect abdominal fluid for amylase and lipase determination.

53. Amylase = 16,000 units/dl; Lipase = 1200 units/dl.

54. Collect pre- and postprandial blood samples for bile acid determination.

54. Preprandial = 5 μmol/L; postprandial = 10 μmol/L.

55. Ultrasound the abdomen.

55. Large gallbladder; normal liver; normal kidneys; hypoechoic, enlarged pancreas.

56. Anesthetize the dog for an exploratory laparotomy.

56. The procedure is aborted when the dog develops refractory hypotension under anesthesia.

Go to Section E

Section E:

Which course of action would you take? *(Choose only one.)*

57. Prescribe thyroid hormone replacement therapy and schedule a recheck in 6 weeks.

57. End of problem.

58. Administer subcutaneous fluids and send the dog home with instructions to feed it a bland diet.

58. End of problem.

59. Begin insulin therapy at a dosage of 0.5 units regular insulin intramuscularly three times daily and monitor blood glucose concentrations.

59. End of problem.

60. Prescribe fenbendazole for 3 days and schedule a recheck examination in 1 month.

60. End of problem.

61. Administer intravenous fluids and allow the dog nothing orally until the vomiting resolves.

61. End of problem.

62. Prescribe an antiemetic and a bland diet with instructions to return the next day if there is no improvement.

62. End of problem.

63. Prescribe prednisone and a mineralocorticoid and recheck in 1 week.

63. End of problem.

END OF PROBLEM

Opening Scene:

The owner of a 6-month-old male Siamese cat presents her cat to you at your rural mixed animal practice in the midwestern United States with a problem of weight loss. He weighed 2 kg at the time of his vaccinations at 4 months of age. Now he weighs 0.8 kg. He hasn't eaten well for the past month and he's not grooming himself. He is an indoor and outdoor cat. He is current on his vaccinations, including rabies.

Go to Section A

Section A:

What questions would you like to ask the owner? *(Choose only the questions you believe relevant to managing the case at this point.)*

1. Is there any possibility of injury or traumatic incident?

2. Do you have any information on his littermates?

3. Do you have other animals?

4. Is he on any medications?

5. Has he had any previous illnesses, injuries, or surgeries?

6. Has he exhibited any difficulty breathing?

7. Has there been any ocular or nasal discharge?

8. Has he seemed less playful or active recently?

9. Has there been any change in your cat's thirst or urination habits?

10. Has your cat vomited or had diarrhea recently?

11. Has your cat collapsed or had any seizures?

12. Has your cat had any changes in mental attitude or personality?

13. What diet is your cat receiving and how much is he fed?

14. Has your cat been treated for intestinal parasites?

1. "It's very unlikely."

2. "I know another one died last month but I don't know why."

3. "Yes, we have six other cats but all are healthy."

4. "No."

5. "No."

6. "No."

7. "No."

8. "Yes, he just lays around and sleeps most of the time or hides."

9. "No changes."

10. "No."

11. "Not that I have seen."

12. "Yes, he seems very depressed."

13. "He used to eat a high quality commercial kitten food free choice, but we have offered him canned food recently to pick up his appetite. He only eats about a tablespoon a day now."

14. "Not that we know of."

Go to Section B

Section B:

Which physical examination procedures would you perform at this time? *(Choose only the procedures you believe relevant to managing the case at this point.)*

15. Measure the rectal body temperature.

15. 39.9°C.

16. Take the pulse and heart rate.

16. The heart rate is 200 beats per minute; the pulse is strong and regular.

17. Measure the respiratory rate and note the character of respirations.

17. The respiratory rate is 16 per minute.

18. Auscultate the lungs.

18. Lung sounds are normal.

19. Auscultate the heart.

19. Heart sounds are normal.

20. Examine the oral cavity.

20. Mucous membranes are pink and moist; capillary refill time is 1 second.

21. Palpate the peripheral lymph nodes.

21. Normal.

22. Palpate the abdomen.

22. The abdomen is distended and feels "doughy."

23. Examine the skin.

23. The hair coat is oily and unkempt; the skin is flaky.

24. Examine the ears, eyes, and nose.

24. No abnormalities.

25. Perform ballottement on the abdomen.

25. A fluid wave is detected.

26. Assess cranial nerves, mental status, postural and spinal reflexes, gait and proprioception.

26. Normal.

27. Palpate the muscles and bones, and flex and extend the joints.

27. Normal.

28. Perform a funduscopic examination.

28. The funduscopic exam is normal.

Go to Section C

Section C:

Which diagnostic procedures would you perform? *(Choose only the procedures you believe relevant to managing the case at this point.)*

29. Collect blood for a complete blood count.

29. The complete blood count results show the following:
PCV = 22%
Hb = 10.2 g/dl
RBC = 6.5 million/mm^3
MCV = 42 fl
MCHC = 33 g/dl

MCH = 15 pg
WBC = 14,800/mm^3
Segs = 11,800/mm^3
Bands = 0/mm^3
Lymphocytes = 1200/mm^3
Monocytes = 1600/mm^3
Eosinophils = 200/mm^3
Basophils = 0/mm^3
Platelets = 245,000/mm^3
Total protein = 9.5 g/dl

30. Collect blood for a serum chemistry profile.

30. The serum chemistry profile results show the following:
Glucose = 143 mg/dl
BUN = 11 mg/dl
Creatinine = 0.6 mg/dl
Albumin = 2.5 g/dl
Total protein = 9.2 g/dl
ALT = 126 IU/L
GGT = 1 IU/L
SAP = 65 IU/L
Amylase = 250 IU/L
Cholesterol = 100 mg/dl
Sodium = 145 mEq/L
Potassium = 3.4 mEq/L
Chloride = 112 mEq/L
Calcium = 9.6 mg/dl
Phosphorous = 3.6 mg/dl
Total bilirubin = 1.5 mg/dl
Total CO_2 = 20 mmol/L

31. Collect urine for a urinalysis.

31. The urine was collected by cystocentesis.
Color = dark yellow
Character = clear
Specific gravity = 1.058
pH = 6.5
Protein = negative
Glucose = negative
Ketones = negative
Bilirubin = 2+
Urobilinogen = negative
Blood = negative
WBC = 1-3/hpf
RBC = 3-5/hpf
Epithelial cells/hpf = occasionally
Bacteria = negative
Casts = negative
Crystals = 1+struvite
Sperm = negative
Fat = negative

32. Collect blood for a feline leukemia virus test.

32. Negative.

33. Collect blood for a feline immunodeficiency virus test.

33. Negative.

34. Perform an abdominal paracentesis for collection of abdominal fluid.

34. Fluid is easily obtained. It is straw-colored. The total protein of the fluid is 5.8 g/dl; the cell count is 1500/mm^3 with nondegenerate neutrophils and mesothelial cells predominating.

35. Collect blood for *Toxoplasma gondii* serology.

35. IgG = 0, IgM = 0.

36. Collect feces for a fecal flotation.

36. *Toxascaris leonina* eggs present.

37. Obtain chest radiographs.

37. Normal.

38. Obtain abdominal radiographs.

38. Lack of abdominal detail precludes interpretation.

39. Perform an echocardiogram.

39. Normal.

40. Collect blood for a feline infectious peritonitis virus test.

40. 1:3200.

Go to Section D

Section D:

Considering the information you have gained so far, what further diagnostic tests would you like to perform? (*Choose only the tests you believe relevant to managing the case at this point.*)

41. Anesthetize the cat and perform a mesenteric angiogram.

41. Normal.

42. Perform a caudal vena cavagram.

42. Normal.

43. Collect fasted and postprandial blood samples for serum bile acid determination.

43. Fasting serum bile acids = 2 µmol/L; postprandial serum bile acids = 5 µmol/L.

44. Ultrasound the abdomen.

44. Large amount of free abdominal fluid is present; intraabdominal organs are normal.

45. Perform an ultrasound-guided liver biopsy.

45. Mild pyogranulomatous hepatitis.

46. Anesthetize the cat to obtain intestinal biopsies by endoscopy.

46. Normal gross appearance of stomach and small intestine; biopsies are pending.

47. Collect aqueous humor by aqueocentesis.

47. Normal.

48. Fast the cat and collect a blood sample for trypsinlike immunoreactivity assay.

48. Results pending.

49. Anesthetize the cat and perform an exploratory laparotomy.

49. The cat suffers a cardiac arrest under anesthesia and cannot be revived.

Section E:

Which course of action would you take? *(Choose only one.)*

50. Prescribe a 21-day course of high-dose clindamycin.

50. End of problem.

51. Prescribe treatment for intestinal parasites, including tapeworms, and recheck the cat in 2 weeks.

51. End of problem.

52. Recommend surgery to correct the portocaval anomaly.

52. End of problem.

53. Inform the owner that the cat has a poor prognosis due to a congenital cardiac defect that cannot be corrected surgically.

53. End of problem.

54. Inform the owner that the cat has probable feline infectious peritonitis virus infection and has a guarded to poor prognosis.

54. End of problem.

55. Prescribe pancreatic enzyme replacement on the food; recheck in 2 weeks.

55. End of problem.

END OF PROBLEM

Opening Scene:

The owner of a 2-year-old neutered male Labrador retriever presents the dog to you with a complaint that the dog is drinking an excessive amount of water. Also, he has urinated in the house a couple of times, which is very unusual for him. He is an indoor dog that has access to a fenced backyard. He lives in the midwestern United States and has not traveled. He is current on his vaccinations, including rabies, and is on monthly heartworm preventative.

Go to Section A

Section A:

What questions would you like to ask the owner? *(Choose only the questions you believe relevant to managing the case at this point.)*

1. Can you estimate how much your dog is drinking?

2. Does he seem to have any difficulty urinating?

3. Is your dog weak or has he ever collapsed?

4. What does he normally eat and how is his appetite?

5. Has he had any previous illnesses, injuries, or surgeries?

6. Has there been any blood in his urine?

7. Does he vomit or have diarrhea?

8. Has there been any hair loss or other skin problems?

9. Has he lost any weight?

10. Is your dog on any medications other than heartworm preventative?

11. What were the circumstances when he urinated in the house?

12. Has your dog had any changes in mental attitude or personality?

13. Do you have any other pets?

14. Has your dog ever had a seizure?

1. "No, I really can't but he seems to drink constantly."

2. "No."

3. "He seems to shake or shiver more when he's standing up."

4. "He eats high protein food normally but he hasn't been cleaning his dish lately."

5. "No, just his neuter at 6 months of age."

6. "Not that I've noticed."

7. "He did vomit twice the other day but I didn't think much about it until you asked."

8. "No."

9. "He has lost a couple pounds."

10. "No."

11. "It was after we had been gone for several hours. He just seemed like he couldn't hold it."

12. "His attitude is a little off for him; he's not as playful as he usually is."

13. "Nope."

14. "Not that we've seen."

Go to Section B

Section B:

Which physical examination procedures would you perform at this time? *(Choose only the procedures you believe relevant to managing the case at this point.)*

15. Measure the body weight.	15. 30 kg.
16. Measure the rectal body temperature.	16. 38.9°C.
17. Take the pulse and heart rate.	17. The heart rate is 108 beats per minute; the pulse is strong and regular.
18. Measure the respiratory rate and note the character of respirations.	18. The respiratory rate is 24 per minute.
19. Auscultate the lungs.	19. Lung sounds are normal.
20. Auscultate the heart.	20. Heart sounds are normal.
21. Examine the oral cavity.	21. The oral cavity is normal; mucous membranes are pink; capillary refill time is 1 second.
22. Palpate the peripheral lymph nodes.	22. The prescapular and submandibular lymph nodes are mildly enlarged and firmer than normal.
23. Palpate the abdomen.	23. Normal.
24. Examine the skin.	24. Normal.
25. Examine the ears, eyes, and nose.	25. No abnormalities.
26. Examine the neck and throat area.	26. Normal.
27. Assess cranial nerves, mental status, postural and spinal reflexes, gait and proprioception.	27. The dog is neurologically normal.
28. Palpate the muscles and bones, and flex and extend the joints.	28. The musculoskeletal system is normal.

Go to Section C

Section C:

Which diagnostic procedures would you perform? *(Choose only the procedures you believe relevant to managing the case at this point.)*

29. Collect blood for a complete blood count.	29. The complete blood count results show the following: PCV = 32% Hb = 12.2 g/dl RBC = 6.5 million/mm^3 MCV = 68 fl MCHC = 32 g/dl

MCH = 23 pg
WBC = 11,800/mm^3
Segs = 9800/mm^3
Bands = 0/mm^3
Lymphocytes = 1200/mm^3
Monocytes = 600/mm^3
Eosinophils = 200/mm^3
Basophils = 0/mm^3
Platelets = 245,000/mm^3
Total protein = 6.5 g/dl

30. Collect blood for a serum BUN and creatinine.

30. BUN = 56 mg/dl
Creatinine = 2.4 mg/dl

31. Collect blood for liver enzyme analysis.

31. ALT = 60 IU/L
GGT = 1 IU/L
SAP = 65 IU/L

32. Collect blood for serum total protein and albumin measurement.

32. Albumin = 3.5 g/dl
Total protein = 6.5 g/dl

33. Collect blood for serum calcium and phosphorus measurement.

33. Calcium = 13.6 mg/dl
Phosphorus = 5.6 mg/dl

34. Collect blood for serum amylase and lipase determination.

34. Amylase = 250 IU/L
Lipase = 100 IU/L

35. Collect blood for serum electrolyte quantitation.

35. Sodium = 145 mEq/L
Potassium = 4.4 mEq/L
Chloride = 112 mEq/L

36. Collect blood for serum blood glucose measurement.

36. Glucose = 105 mg/dl.

37. Collect blood for serum cholesterol measurement.

37. Cholesterol = 100 mg/dl.

38. Collect blood for serum bilirubin determination.

38. Total bilirubin = 0.1 mg/dl.

39. Collect urine for a complete urinalysis.

39. The urine was collected by cystocentesis.
Color = yellow
Character = clear
Specific gravity = 1.007
pH = 6.5
Protein = negative
Glucose = negative
Ketones = negative
Bilirubin = 1+
Urobilinogen = negative
Blood = negative
WBC = 1-3/hpf
RBC = 3-5/hpf
Epithelial cells/hpf = occasionally
Bacteria = negative
Casts = occasional coarse granular casts

Crystals = 1+ calcium oxalate
Sperm = negative
Fat = negative

40. Measure 24-hour water consumption.

40. 125 ml/kg/24 hr.

41. Perform a fine needle aspiration biopsy of the lymph nodes.

41. Consistent with but not diagnostic for histiocytic lymphoma.

42. Collect urine for aerobic bacterial culture and antibiotic sensitivity.

42. Negative.

43. Collect blood before and 3 and 8 hours after giving the dog 0.015 mg/kg dexamethasone intravenously for serum cortisol determination.

43. 0 hr = 3.5 μg/dl; 3 hr = 0.9 μg/dl; 8 hr = 0.5 μg/dl.

44. Palpate the dog's prostate.

44. Normal.

Go to Section D

Section D:

Considering the information you have gained so far, what further diagnostic tests would you like to perform? (*Choose only the tests you believe relevant to managing the case at this point.*)

45. Perform a 24-hour creatinine clearance.

45. 1.8 ml/kg/min.

46. Obtain radiographs of the abdomen.

46. Normal.

47. Obtain radiographs of the chest.

47. Normal.

48. Sedate the dog and collect a sample of bone marrow from the wing of the ilium.

48. Normal.

49. Ultrasound the abdomen.

49. No abnormal findings.

50. Collect blood for a serum parathyroid hormone assay.

50. Results pending.

51. Palpate the dog's rectum and perianal area.

51. No abnormal findings.

52. Perform a water deprivation test.

52. The dog begins vomiting after 4 hours, and the test is aborted.

53. Anesthetize the dog and remove a prescapular lymph node for biopsy.

53. Results pending.

54. Perform an intravenous pyelogram.

54. Normal nephrogram, mild delay in dye clearance.

55. Collect blood pre- and post-ACTH administration for serum cortisol determination.

55. Pre-ACTH cortisol = 3.4 μg/dl; post-ACTH cortisol = 14.1 μg/dl.

56. Anesthetize the dog for a renal biopsy.

56. Results pending.

Section E:

Which course of action would you take? *(Choose only one.)*

57. Prescribe oral prednisone at a dose of 1.0 mg/kg daily and recheck the serum chemistry panel.

57. End of problem.

58. Place the dog on intravenous 0.9% NaCl and furosemide until the lymph node biopsies are received.

58. End of problem.

59. Perform a surgical exploration of the neck for parathyroid neoplasia.

59. End of problem.

60. Institute induction therapy with o,p'-DDD and recheck the dog in 2 weeks.

60. End of problem.

61. Send the dog home with instructions for the owner to restrict the dog's water intake to 75% of what he was drinking and have them bring him back in 1 week for a recheck urinalysis.

61. End of problem.

62. Prescribe a protein-restricted diet and give the owners a poor prognosis.

62. End of problem.

END OF PROBLEM

Opening Scene:

The owner of a 9-year-old spayed female domestic shorthaired cat presents her cat to you at your specialty cat practice with a problem of increased thirst and urination of 4 weeks duration. The cat's appetite is very good, but she has lost about 1 kg of body weight. The cat is always indoors. She is current on her vaccinations, including rabies.

Go to Section A

Section A:

What questions would you like to ask the owner? *(Choose only the questions you believe relevant to managing the case at this point.)*

1. Can you estimate how much your cat drinks?

1. "No, I really don't know, although I see her drinking all the time from the toilet, the drippy faucet, and even the dog's bowl."

2. Does she urinate more frequently or just in larger volumes?

2. "She does go a little more frequently, but mostly it's large volumes at a time. I have to change the litter box daily."

3. Does she appear to have any pain associated with urination?

3. "No."

4. Does she use her litter box appropriately?

4. "Yes."

5. Has she had any previous illnesses, injuries, or surgeries?

5. "No, only her spay surgery at 6 months of age."

6. What is her diet and how much does she eat daily?

6. "She eats three cans of commercial canned cat food a day and always meows for more."

7. Is she on any medications?

7. "No."

8. Has your cat been vomiting or had any diarrhea?

8. "No."

9. Do you have other animals?

9. "Yes, we have a dog, too."

10. Does your cat appear to be lame?

10. "No."

11. Has your cat collapsed or had any seizures?

11. "Not that I have seen."

12. Has your cat had any changes in mental attitude or personality?

12. "Her attitude is great."

13. Does your cat have any skin disease?

13. "No."

Section B:

Which physical examination procedures would you perform at this time? *(Choose only the procedures you believe relevant to managing the case at this point.)*

14. Measure the rectal body temperature.

15. Take the pulse and heart rate.

16. Measure the respiratory rate and note the character of respirations.

17. Auscultate the lungs.

18. Auscultate the heart.

19. Examine the oral cavity.

20. Palpate the peripheral lymph nodes.

21. Palpate the abdomen.

22. Examine the skin.

23. Examine the ears, eyes, and nose.

24. Assess the hydration status.

25. Assess cranial nerves, mental status, postural and spinal reflexes, gait and proprioception.

26. Palpate the muscles and bones, and flex and extend the joints.

27. Palpate the neck.

14. 38.3°C.

15. The heart rate is 144 beats per minute; the pulse is strong and regular.

16. The respiratory rate is 16 per minute.

17. Lung sounds are normal.

18. Heart sounds are normal.

19. Mild dental tartar; mucous membranes are pink; capillary refill time is 1 second.

20. Normal.

21. Normal except for slight hepatomegaly.

22. Normal.

23. No abnormalities.

24. Normal.

25. The cat is neurologically normal.

26. The musculoskeletal system is normal.

27. No abnormalities.

Go to Section C

Section C:

Which diagnostic procedures would you perform? *(Choose only the procedures you believe relevant to managing the case at this point.)*

28. Collect blood for a complete blood count.

28. The complete blood count results show the following:
PCV = 42%
Hb = 18.2 g/dl
RBC = 11.5 million/mm^3
MCV = 42 fl
MCHC = 33 g/dl
MCH = 15 pg

WBC = 14,800/mm^3
Segs = 11,800/mm^3
Bands = 0/mm^3
Lymphocytes = 1800/mm^3
Monocytes = 1000/mm^3
Eosinophils = 200/mm^3
Basophils = 0/mm^3
Platelets = 245,000/mm^3
Total protein = 6.5 g/dl

29. Collect blood for a serum glucose concentration.

29. Glucose = 405 mg/dl

30. Collect blood for BUN and creatinine determination.

30. BUN = 26 mg/dl
Creatinine = 1.6 mg/dl

31. Collect blood for serum liver enzyme measurement.

31. ALT = 260 IU/L
GGT = 3 IU/L
SAP = 165 IU/L

32. Collect blood for calcium and phosphorus determination.

32. Calcium = 9.6 mg/dl
Phosphorus = 3.6 mg/dl

33. Collect blood for serum cholesterol measurement.

33. Cholesterol = 324 mg/dl.

34. Collect blood for arterial blood gas analysis.

34. The results of the arterial blood gas analysis show the following:
pH = 7.35
pCO$_2$ = 30 mm Hg
pO$_2$ = 95 mm Hg
HCO$_3$ = 18 mg/dl

35. Collect blood for a serum thyroid hormone concentration.

35. Serum thyroxine = 2.0 μg/dl.

36. Collect urine for a urinalysis.

36. The urine was collected by cystocentesis.
Color = yellow
Character = clear
Specific gravity = 1.028
pH = 6.5
Protein = negative
Glucose = 4+
Ketones = negative
Bilirubin = negative
Urobilinogen = negative
Blood = negative
WBC = 1-3/hpf
RBC = 3-5/hpf
Epithelial cells/hpf = occasionally
Bacteria = negative
Casts = negative
Crystals = negative
Sperm = negative
Fat = negative

37. Collect blood for a feline leukemia virus test.

37. Negative.

| 38. | Collect blood for a feline immunodeficiency virus test. | 38. | Negative. |

38. Collect blood for a feline immunodeficiency virus test.

38. Negative.

39. Collect urine for an aerobic bacterial culture and antimicrobial sensitivity.

39. No growth.

40. Obtain chest radiographs.

40. Normal.

41. Obtain abdominal radiographs.

41. Normal except for mild diffuse hepatomegaly.

42. Quantitate 24 hour water intake.

42. The cat drank 110 ml/kg/24 hours.

43. Perform a water deprivation test.

43. The cat's urine concentrated to a specific gravity of 1.042 as it became 5% dehydrated.

44. Administer 0.5 units antidiuretic hormone/kg intramuscularly and measure urine specific gravity at 30, 60, and 120 minutes post-injection.

44. The cat's urine concentration increased to 1.078.

Go to Section D

Section D:

Considering the information you have gained so far, what further diagnostic tests would you like to perform? *(Choose only the tests you believe relevant to managing the case at this point.)*

45. Collect blood for a serum insulin concentration.

45. Results pending.

46. Collect blood for a serum trypsinlike immunoreactivity assay.

46. Results pending.

47. Collect blood before and 3 and 8 hours after 0.015 mg/kg dexamethasone is given intravenously for serum cortisol determination.

47. 0 hr cortisol = 3.9 µg/dl; 3 hr cortisol = 0.4 µg/dl; 8 hr cortisol = 0.3 µg/dl.

48. Perform a funduscopic examination.

48. Normal.

49. Collect fasting and postprandial blood samples for serum bile acid analysis.

49. Fasting serum bile acids = 3 mmol/L; postprandial serum bile acids = 5 mmol/L.

50. Ultrasound the abdomen.

50. Diffuse increase in echogenicity to the liver, which is generally enlarged. No other abnormalities.

51. Collect blood for feline infectious peritonitis virus serology.

51. 1:100.

52. Collect blood for *Toxoplasma* serology.

52. IgG = 1:4; IgM = 1:4.

53. Anesthetize the cat for upper gastrointestinal endoscopy.

53. No gross abnormalities; biopsies pending.

54. Refer the cat to a specialist for a computerized tomogram of the brain.

54. No abnormal findings.

55. Perform a 24-hour creatinine clearance.

55. Normal.

Go to Section E

Section E:

Which course of action would you take? *(Choose only one.)*

56. Prescribe methimazole and schedule a recheck examination in 2 weeks.

56. End of problem.

57. Initiate insulin therapy with 1 unit of lente insulin subcutaneously twice daily.

57. End of problem.

58. Prescribe 6 weeks of cephalexin and schedule a recheck examination in 2 weeks.

58. End of problem.

59. Recommend euthanasia because the prognosis for liver disease is poor.

59. End of problem.

60. Sign the cat up for radiation therapy for a pituitary tumor.

60. End of problem.

61. Put the cat on the waiting list for radioactive iodine therapy.

61. End of problem.

62. Prescribe ketoconazole and reevaluate the cat in 1 week.

62. End of problem.

END OF PROBLEM

Opening Scene:

The owner of a 3-month-old female Miniature pinscher presents the dog to you at your small animal practice with complaints that the puppy is not gaining weight adequately and has seemed listless over the past week. Her appetite seems good, and at times she is very playful. She lives in the western United States and has not traveled. She has had her first two distemper/parvovirus combination vaccinations and is due for another booster in 3 weeks.

Go to Section A

Section A:

What questions would you like to ask the owner? (*Choose only the questions you believe relevant to managing the case at this point.*)

1. Has she had any previous illnesses, injuries, or surgeries?

1. "No."

2. Has there been any change in her thirst or urinary habits?

2. "She does seem to drink a lot but I thought it was because she is a puppy."

3. Has there been any blood in her urine or evidence of difficult urination?

3. "No."

4. What does she normally eat and how is her appetite?

4. "She eats a high quality puppy food—all that I give her, which is one-fourth cup three times daily."

5. Is your dog weak or has she ever collapsed?

5. "No."

6. Does the listlessness worsen after eating?

6. "Now that you mention it, that's when she's the most listless."

7. Does she vomit or have diarrhea?

7. "She does vomit and have a loose stool occasionally, but not frequently enough to have concerned me."

8. Are you missing any of her toys?

8. "Not that I'm aware of."

9. Has she been tested or treated for intestinal parasites?

9. "No."

10. Is there any possibility of toxin exposure?

10. "No."

11. Has there been any recent trauma?

11. "No."

12. Other than the listlessness, has your dog had any changes in mental attitude or personality?

12. "She just gets listless usually, but actually, she did get a little aggressive one time."

13. Do you have any other pets?

13. "Nope."

14. Has your dog ever had a seizure?

14. "Not that we've seen."

Go to Section B

Section B:

Which physical examination procedures would you perform at this time? *(Choose only the procedures you believe relevant to managing the case at this point.)*

15. Measure the body weight.

16. Measure the rectal body temperature.

17. Take the pulse and heart rate.

18. Measure the respiratory rate and note the character of respirations.

19. Auscultate the lungs.

20. Auscultate the heart.

21. Examine the oral cavity.

22. Palpate the peripheral lymph nodes.

23. Palpate the abdomen.

24. Examine the skin.

25. Examine the ears, eyes, and nose.

26. Examine the neck and throat area.

27. Assess cranial nerves, mental status, postural and spinal reflexes, gait and proprioception.

28. Palpate the muscles and bones, and flex and extend the joints.

15. 1.2 kg.

16. 38.9°C.

17. The heart rate is 168 beats per minute; the pulse is strong and regular.

18. The respiratory rate is 24 per minute.

19. Lung sounds are normal.

20. Heart sounds are normal.

21. The oral cavity is normal; mucous membranes are pink; capillary refill time is 1 second.

22. Normal.

23. Normal.

24. Normal.

25. No abnormalities.

26. Normal.

27. The dog is neurologically normal.

28. The musculoskeletal system is normal.

Go to Section C

Section C:

Which diagnostic procedures would you perform? *(Choose only the procedures you believe relevant to managing the case at this point.)*

29. Collect blood for a complete blood count.

29. The complete blood count results show the following:
PCV = 32%
Hb = 12.2 g/dl
RBC = 6.5 million/mm^3
MCV = 59 fl
MCHC = 32 g/dl
MCH = 23 pg

WBC = 11,800/mm^3
Segs = 9800/mm^3
Bands = 0/mm^3
Lymphocytes = 1200/mm^3
Monocytes = 600/mm^3
Eosinophils = 200/mm^3
Basophils = 0/mm^3
Platelets = 245,000/mm^3
Total protein = 4.0 g/dl

30. Collect blood for a serum BUN and creatinine.

30. BUN = 8 mg/dl
Creatinine = 0.6 mg/dl

31. Collect blood for liver enzyme analysis.

31. ALT = 60 IU/L
GGT = 1 IU/L
SAP = 265 IU/L

32. Collect blood for serum total protein and albumin measurement.

32. Albumin = 2.3 g/dl
Total protein = 4.0 g/dl

33. Collect blood for serum calcium and phosphorus measurement.

33. Calcium = 12.6 mg/dl
Phosphorus = 8.6 mg/dl

34. Collect blood for serum amylase and lipase determination.

34. Amylase = 250 IU/L
Lipase = 100 IU/L

35. Collect blood for serum electrolyte quantitation.

35. Sodium = 145 mEq/L
Potassium = 4.4 mEq/L
Chloride = 112 mEq/L

36. Collect blood for serum blood glucose measurement.

36. Glucose = 105 mg/dl

37. Collect blood for serum cholesterol measurement.

37. Cholesterol = 100 mg/dl

38. Collect blood for serum bilirubin determination.

38. Total bilirubin = 0.1 mg/dl

39. Collect urine for a complete urinalysis.

39. The urine was collected by cystocentesis.
Color = yellow
Character = clear
Specific gravity = 1.007
pH = 7.5
Protein = negative
Glucose = negative
Ketones = negative
Bilirubin = 1+
Urobilinogen = negative
Blood = negative
WBC = 0-1/hpf
RBC = 3-5/hpf
Epithelial cells/hpf = occasionally
Bacteria = negative
Casts = negative
Crystals = 1+ammonium biurate
Sperm = negative
Fat = negative

40. Collect stool for fecal flotation.

41. Obtain chest radiographs.

42. Obtain abdominal radiographs.

43. Collect blood for lead analysis.

44. Collect blood for a canine distemper titer.

40. *Toxocara canis* ova present.

41. Normal.

42. Lack of detail precludes interpretation; however, it can be stated that the liver size is markedly reduced.

43. 0.2 ppm (normal<0.35 ppm).

44. 1:2.

Go to Section D

Section D:

Considering the information you have gained so far, what further diagnostic tests would you like to perform? (*Choose only the tests you believe relevant to managing the case at this point.*)

45. Collect blood for fasting and postprandial serum bile acids determination.

46. Collect blood before and after giving an ammonia solution orally for blood ammonia measurement.

47. Anesthetize the dog for cerebrospinal fluid collection.

48. Collect cerebrospinal fluid under anesthesia for canine distemper antibody assay.

49. Perform an echocardiogram.

50. Collect blood for trypsinlike immunoreactivity assay.

51. Anesthetize the dog and perform an exploratory laparotomy.

52. Perform a water deprivation test.

53. Ultrasound the abdomen.

54. Anesthetize the dog for portal angiography.

55. Collect blood pre- and post-ACTH administration for serum cortisol determination.

56. Refer the dog to a specialist for computerized tomography of the brain.

45. Fasting serum bile acids = 85 mmol/L; post-prandial serum bile acids = 236 mmol/L.

46. Resting blood ammonia = 100 µg/dl; post challenge value not available because the dog vomited.

47. Normal.

48. CSF canine distemper titer = 0.

49. No abnormal findings.

50. Results pending.

51. Small liver; biopsies pending.

52. Her urine is concentrated to 1.025 after 6 hours of water deprivation.

53. The liver is small; no other abnormalities are noted.

54. A single intrahepatic portal-venous anomaly is identified.

55. Pre-ACTH cortisol = 3.4 µg/dl; post-ACTH cortisol = 14.1 µg/dl.

56. No abnormalities.

Section E:

Which course of action would you take? *(Choose only one.)*

57. Prescribe an anthelmintic and a high protein diet and advise the owner to weigh the puppy at weekly intervals.

57. End of problem.

58. Prescribe pancreatic enzyme replacement and recheck the puppy in 2 weeks.

58. End of problem.

59. Recommend that the owners accept referral to a surgeon for ligation of the portocaval anomaly.

59. End of problem.

60. Diagnose canine distemper and recommend euthanasia.

60. End of problem.

61. Refer the dog to a specialist for further workup.

61. End of problem.

62. Prescribe a protein-restricted diet and give the owners a poor prognosis.

62. End of problem.

END OF PROBLEM

Opening Scene:

The owner of a 5-year-old neutered male domestic shorthaired cat presents her cat to you with a problem of hemorrhagic nasal discharge of 2 day's duration. It began the night before last after an episode of sneezing. He bled for an hour or so, then it stopped spontaneously. Since then he has had an intermittent, mild bloody discharge. He is an indoor and outdoor cat. He is current on his vaccinations, including rabies.

Go to Section A

Section A:

What questions would you like to ask the owner? (*Choose only the questions you believe relevant to managing the case at this point.*)

1. Has your cat been sneezing other than the night before last?

2. Is the discharge unilateral or bilateral?

3. Is he bleeding anywhere else that you know of?

4. Is there a possibility of toxin exposure?

5. Has he had any previous illnesses, injuries, or surgeries?

6. What is his diet and how much does he eat daily?

7. Is he on any medications?

8. Has your cat been vomiting or had any diarrhea?

9. Do you have other animals?

10. Has there been any change in his thirst or urination habits?

11. Has your cat collapsed or had any seizures?

12. Has your cat had any changes in mental attitude or personality?

13. Does your cat have any skin disease?

1. "He has sneezed just two or three times over the past 2 days."

2. "I don't really know."

3. "Not that I've seen."

4. "Well, he goes outside and I don't really know what he could get into."

5. "No, only his neuter surgery at a year of age."

6. "He eats dry commercial cat food, about one-half cup a day."

7. "No."

8. "No."

9. "Yes, we have three other cats, too."

10. "No."

11. "Not that I have seen."

12. "His attitude is a little off; maybe he's a bit quiet for him."

13. "No."

Section B:

Which physical examination procedures would you perform at this time? *(Choose only the procedures you believe relevant to managing the case at this point.)*

14. Measure the body weight.

14. 4.5 kg.

15. Measure the rectal body temperature.

15. 38.3°C.

16. Take the pulse and heart rate.

16. The heart rate is 144 beats per minute; the pulse is strong and regular.

17. Measure the respiratory rate and note the character of respirations.

17. The respiratory rate is 16 per minute.

18. Auscultate the lungs.

18. Lung sounds are normal.

19. Auscultate the heart.

19. Heart sounds are normal.

20. Examine the oral cavity.

20. Mild gingivitis; mucous membranes are pink; capillary refill time is 1 second.

21. Palpate the peripheral lymph nodes.

21. Normal.

22. Palpate the abdomen.

22. Normal.

23. Examine the skin.

23. Normal.

24. Examine the ears, eyes, and nose.

24. No abnormalities except for dried blood around the right nostril.

25. Assess the hydration status.

25. Normal.

26. Assess cranial nerves, mental status, postural and spinal reflexes, gait and proprioception.

26. The cat is neurologically normal.

27. Palpate the muscles and bones, and flex and extend the joints.

27. The musculoskeletal system is normal.

28. Palpate the neck.

28. No abnormalities.

Go to Section C

Section C:

Which diagnostic procedures would you perform? *(Choose only the procedures you believe relevant to managing the case at this point.)*

29. Collect blood for a complete blood count.

29. The complete blood count results show the following:
PCV = 42%
Hb = 18.2 g/dl
RBC = 11.5 million/mm^3
MCV = 42 fl

MCHC = 33 g/dl
MCH = 15 pg
WBC = 2800/mm^3
Segs = 800/mm^3
Bands = 0/mm^3
Lymphocytes = 1800/mm^3
Monocytes = 100/mm^3
Eosinophils = 100/mm^3
Basophils = 0/mm^3
Platelets = 10,000/mm^3
Total protein = 8.2 g/dl

30. Collect blood for a serum glucose concentration.

30. Glucose = 105 mg/dl

31. Collect blood for a BUN and creatinine determination.

31. BUN = 46 mg/dl
Creatinine = 1.0 mg/dl

32. Collect blood for serum liver enzyme measurement.

32. ALT = 60 IU/L
GGT = 1 IU/L
SAP = 65 IU/L

33. Collect blood for calcium and phosphorus determination.

33. Calcium = 9.6 mg/dl
Phosphorus = 3.6 mg/dl

34. Collect blood for serum cholesterol measurement.

34. Cholesterol = 124 mg/dl.

35. Collect blood for blood gas analysis.

35. The results of the blood gas analysis show the following:
pH = 7.35
pCO_2 = 30 mm Hg
pO_2 = 95 mm Hg
HCO_3 = 18 mg/dl

36. Collect blood for a serum thyroid hormone concentration.

36. Serum thyroxine = 2.0 µg/dl.

37. Collect urine for a urinalysis.

37. The urine was collected free catch.
Color = yellow
Character = clear
Specific gravity = 1.048
pH = 6.5
Protein = negative
Glucose = negative
Ketones = negative
Bilirubin = negative
Urobilinogen = negative
Blood = 2+
WBC = 1-3/hpf
RBC = 5-10/hpf
Epithelial cells/hpf = occasionally
Bacteria = negative
Casts = negative
Crystals = negative
Sperm = negative
Fat = negative

38. Collect blood for a feline leukemia virus test.

38. Positive.

39. Collect blood for a feline immunodeficiency virus test.

39. Positive.

40. Collect blood for coagulation studies.

40. Prothrombin time = 8 seconds (normal = 6-10 seconds); Activated partial thromboplastin time = 10 seconds (normal = 12-18 seconds); Activated clotting time = 130 seconds (normal = 60-120 seconds); Platelet count = 10,000/mm^3.

41. Obtain chest radiographs.

41. Normal.

42. Obtain abdominal radiographs.

42. Normal.

43. Measure systolic and diastolic blood pressures.

43. Systolic blood pressure = 145 mm Hg; diastolic blood pressure = 85 mm Hg.

44. Anesthetize the cat for skull radiographs.

44. Soft tissue density in right nasal cavity; no other lesions.

45. Collect a nasal discharge sample for cytology.

45. Consistent with hemorrhage.

Go to Section D

Section D:

Considering the information you have gained so far, what further diagnostic tests would you like to perform? *(Choose only the tests you believe relevant to managing the case at this point.)*

46. Collect blood for *Cryptococcus neoformans* serology.

46. Results pending.

47. Collect blood for an antinuclear antibody titer.

47. The antinuclear antibody titer is 1:20.

48. Anesthetize the cat for the collection of bone marrow.

48. No megakaryocytes present; maturation arrest of myeloid precursors; M:E = 0.5:1.2.

49. Perform a funduscopic examination.

49. Mild petechial retinal hemorrhages bilaterally; otherwise normal.

50. Collect fasting and postprandial blood samples for serum bile acid analysis.

50. Fasting serum bile acids = 3 mmol/L; post-prandial serum bile acids = 5 mmol/L.

51. Ultrasound the abdomen.

51. Normal.

52. Collect blood for feline infectious peritonitis virus serology.

52. 1:100.

53. Collect blood for *Toxoplasma* serology.

53. IgG = 1:4; IgM = 1:4.

54. Collect blood for a T$_3$ suppression test.

54. The T$_4$ before T$_3$ administration was 2.0 µg/dl. The T$_4$ following administration of T$_3$ was 0.5 µg/dl (normal<1.5 µg/dl). The serum T$_3$ measured to confirm administration of the T$_3$ increased appropriately.

55. Anesthetize the cat for a rhinoscopic examination and nasal biopsies.

55. No gross abnormalities other than hemorrhage; biopsies pending.

56. Perform an echocardiogram.

56. Normal.

Go to Section E

Section E:

Which course of action would you take? *(Choose only one.)*

57. Prescribe methimazole and schedule a recheck examination in 2 weeks.

57. End of problem.

58. Schedule the cat for radiation therapy for a nasal tumor.

58. End of problem.

59. Prescribe 6 weeks of cephalexin and schedule a recheck examination in 2 weeks.

59. End of problem.

60. Administer a whole blood transfusion and send the cat home.

60. End of problem.

61. Prescribe propranolol and recheck the cat in 1 week.

61. End of problem.

62. Advise the owners of the poor prognosis and recommend euthanasia.

62. End of problem.

63. Prescribe ketoconazole and reevaluate the cat in 1 week.

63. End of problem.

64. Prescribe vitamin K1 and recheck the cat in 1 week.

64. End of problem.

END OF PROBLEM

Opening Scene:

The owner of a 2-year-old female Great Dane presents the dog to you with complaints that the dog has had an acute onset of bloody diarrhea. In addition, she has vomited four to five times over the last 24 hours. She has no appetite for anything. She lives in the western United States and has not traveled. She is up to date on her vaccinations, including distemper/parvovirus and rabies and is on monthly heartworm preventative.

Go to Section A

Section A:

What questions would you like to ask the owner? *(Choose only the questions you believe relevant to managing the case at this point.)*

1. Has she had any previous illnesses, injuries, or surgeries?

2. Has there been any change in her thirst or urinary habits?

3. Is she currently taking any medications?

4. What diet does she normally eat and about how much does she consume in a day?

5. Is your dog weak or has she ever collapsed?

6. Could you describe her diarrhea and vomitus?

7. Has she been given table scraps or gotten into the garbage recently?

8. Has she been coughing or sneezing?

9. Has she been tested or treated for intestinal parasites?

10. Is there any possibility of toxin exposure?

11. Has there been any recent trauma?

12. Has your dog had any changes in mental attitude or personality?

13. Do you have any other pets?

14. Has your dog ever had a seizure?

1. "She was spayed at 8 months of age; otherwise she's been normal."

2. "No changes."

3. "No."

4. "She eats a premium dry dog food. She used to easily finish about 6 cups daily, but she hasn't eaten anything since yesterday morning."

5. "She hasn't collapsed but doesn't seem to have her usual get up and go. Also, she trembles when she stands up for long periods of time."

6. "The diarrhea is very watery and red wine in color. It smells awful. She has had diarrhea six times since yesterday afternoon. The vomit is always a yellow foam."

7. "No, we never give her anything other than her dog food and some dog treats. She can't get into the garbage."

8. "No."

9. "No."

10. "No."

11. "No."

12. "No."

13. "Nope."

14. "Not that we've seen."

Go to Section B

Section B:

Which physical examination procedures would you perform at this time? *(Choose only the procedures you believe relevant to managing the case at this point.)*

15. Measure the body weight.

16. Measure the rectal body temperature.

17. Take the pulse and heart rate.

18. Measure the respiratory rate and note the character of respirations.

19. Auscultate the lungs.

20. Auscultate the heart.

21. Examine the oral cavity.

22. Palpate the peripheral lymph nodes.

23. Palpate the abdomen.

24. Assess the hydration status.

25. Examine the ears, eyes, and nose.

26. Examine the neck and throat area.

27. Assess cranial nerves, mental status, postural and spinal reflexes, gait and proprioception.

28. Palpate the muscles and bones, and flex and extend the joints.

15. 50.2 kg.

16. 39.9°C.

17. The heart rate is 168 beats per minute; the pulse is strong and regular.

18. The respiratory rate is 24 per minute.

19. Lung sounds are normal.

20. Heart sounds are normal.

21. The oral cavity is normal; mucous membranes are pink; capillary refill time is 1 second.

22. Normal.

23. The dog seems uncomfortable when the abdomen is palpated.

24. She is 5% dehydrated.

25. No abnormalities.

26. Normal.

27. The dog is neurologically normal.

28. The musculoskeletal system is normal.

Go to Section C

Section C:

Which diagnostic procedures would you perform? *(Choose only the procedures you believe relevant to managing the case at this point.)*

29. Collect blood for a complete blood count.

29. The complete blood count results show the following:
    PCV = 48%
    Hb = 13.2 g/dl
    RBC = 8.5 million/mm^3
    MCV = 68 fl
    MCHC = 32 g/dl

MCH = 23 pg
WBC = 29,000/mm^3
Segs = 25,800/mm^3
Bands = 1200/mm^3
Lymphocytes = 1200/mm^3
Monocytes = 200/mm^3
Eosinophils = 600/mm^3
Basophils = 0/mm^3
Platelets = 245,000/mm^3
Total protein = 8.0 g/dl

30. Collect blood for a serum BUN and creatinine.

30. BUN = 58 mg/dl
Creatinine = 2.6 mg/dl

31. Collect blood for liver enzyme analysis.

31. ALT = 320 IU/L
GGT = 1 IU/L
SAP = 65 IU/L

32. Collect blood for serum total protein and albumin measurement.

32. Albumin = 4.3 g/dl
Total protein = 8.0 g/dl

33. Collect blood for serum calcium and phosphorus measurement.

33. Calcium = 10.6 mg/dl
Phosphorus = 3.6 mg/dl

34. Collect blood for serum amylase and lipase determination.

34. Amylase = 250 IU/L
Lipase = 100 IU/L

35. Collect blood for serum electrolyte quantitation.

35. Sodium = 135 mEq/L
Potassium = 6.4 mEq/L
Chloride = 102 mEq/L

36. Collect blood for serum blood glucose measurement.

36. Glucose = 105 mg/dl

37. Collect blood for serum cholesterol measurement.

37. Cholesterol = 100 mg/dl

38. Collect blood for serum bilirubin determination.

38. Total bilirubin = 0.1 mg/dl

39. Collect urine for a complete urinalysis.

39. The urine was collected by cystocentesis.
Color = yellow
Character = clear
Specific gravity = 1.057
pH = 7.5
Protein = negative
Glucose = negative
Ketones = negative
Bilirubin = negative
Urobilinogen = negative
Blood = negative
WBC = 0-1/hpf
RBC = 3-5/hpf
Epithelial cells/hpf = occasionally
Bacteria = negative
Casts = negative
Crystals = negative
Sperm = negative
Fat = negative

40. Collect stool for fecal flotation.	40. Numerous *Trichuris vulpis* eggs.
41. Obtain chest radiographs.	41. Normal.
42. Obtain abdominal radiographs.	42. Normal.
43. Collect blood for lead analysis.	43. 0.2 ppm (normal<0.35 ppm).
44. Perform an electrocardiogram.	44. Sinus tachycardia.

Go to Section D

Section D:

Considering the information you have gained so far, what further diagnostic tests would you like to perform? (*Choose only the tests you believe relevant to managing the case at this point.*)

45. Collect blood for fasting and postprandial serum bile acids determination.	45. Fasting serum bile acids = 5 mmol/L; post-prandial serum bile acids = 6 mmol/L.
46. Perform an intravenous pyelogram.	46. Normal.
47. Ultrasound the abdomen.	47. Normal.
48. Anesthetize the dog and perform intestinal biopsies by endoscopy.	48. Mucosa of the stomach and small intestine are diffusely reddened; active hemorrhage is noted; biopsies pending.
49. Perform an echocardiogram.	49. No abnormal findings.
50. Collect blood for trypsinlike immunoreactivity assay.	50. Results pending.
51. Anesthetize the dog and perform an exploratory laparotomy.	51. Serosal surface of the intestines is diffusely reddened; biopsies pending.
52. Perform a water deprivation test.	52. She vomits and becomes extremely depressed after 4 hours of water deprivation.
53. Perform a 24-hour creatinine clearance test.	53. 2.0 ml/kg/min.
54. Pass a urinary catheter to determine the patency of the lower urinary tract.	54. Normal.
55. Collect blood pre- and post-ACTH administration for serum cortisol determination.	55. Pre-ACTH cortisol = 6 μg/dl; post-ACTH cortisol = 18.4 μg/dl.
56. Administer barium and perform an upper gastrointestinal radiographic series.	56. Diffuse enteritis; no obstruction noted.

Section E:

Which course of action would you take? *(Choose only one.)*

57. Prescribe a mineralocorticoid and glucocorticoid at physiological dosages and recheck the laboratory values in 6 to 12 hours.

57. End of problem.

58. Administer a whole blood transfusion, followed by intravenous fluid therapy.

58. End of problem.

59. Diagnose parvoviral enteritis and give the owners a poor prognosis.

59. End of problem.

60. Administer an anthelmintic, intravenous antibiotics, and 0.9% saline to replace dehydration losses and to provide maintenance fluids.

60. End of problem.

61. Refer the dog to a specialist for further workup.

61. End of problem.

END OF PROBLEM

Opening Scene:

The owner of an 8-year-old spayed female domestic shorthaired cat presents her cat to you with a problem of anorexia of 2 weeks duration. She usually eats dry cat food. When she quit eating that, the owner tried canned cat foods, which she ate for a few days, although only in small amounts. Now she refuses everything, even chicken livers. She is an indoor cat. She is current on her vaccinations, including rabies.

Go to Section A

Section A:

What questions would you like to ask the owner? (*Choose only the questions you believe relevant to managing the case at this point.*)

1. Has your cat lost weight?

1. "I think so. She used to weigh 6 kg."

2. Have there been any changes in your household, for instance, a new baby, new pets, etc.?

2. "Well, I just got married so there is a new person in the house. Also, we were gone for a week about a month ago on our honeymoon."

3. Has your cat been vomiting or had any diarrhea?

3. "Yes, she has vomited two or three times over the last week."

4. Is there a possibility of toxin exposure?

4. "No."

5. Has she had any previous illnesses, injuries, or surgeries?

5. "No, only her spay surgery at a year of age."

6. Is she on any medications?

6. "No."

7. Do you have other animals?

7. "No."

8. Has she been sneezing or coughing or had any nasal discharge?

8. "No."

9. Has she been lame at all?

9. "No."

10. Has there been any change in her thirst or urination habits?

10. "No."

11. Has your cat collapsed or had any seizures?

11. "Not that I have seen."

12. Has your cat had any changes in mental attitude or personality?

12. "She's very quiet and has started hiding."

13. Does your cat have any skin disease?

13. "No."

Section B:

Which physical examination procedures would you perform at this time? *(Choose only the procedures you believe relevant to managing the case at this point.)*

14. Measure the body weight.

14. 5.2 kg.

15. Measure the rectal body temperature.

15. 38.3°C.

16. Take the pulse and heart rate.

16. The heart rate is 180 beats per minute; the pulse is strong and regular.

17. Measure the respiratory rate and note the character of respirations.

17. The respiratory rate is 16 per minute.

18. Auscultate the lungs.

18. Lung sounds are normal.

19. Auscultate the heart.

19. Heart sounds are normal.

20. Examine the oral cavity.

20. Mucous membranes are orangish pink; capillary refill time is 1 second.

21. Palpate the peripheral lymph nodes.

21. Normal.

22. Palpate the abdomen.

22. The liver is enlarged.

23. Examine the skin.

23. Normal.

24. Examine the ears, eyes, and nose.

24. No abnormalities except the yellowish hue to the skin of the pinnae.

25. Assess the hydration status.

25. Normal.

26. Assess cranial nerves, mental status, postural and spinal reflexes, gait and proprioception.

26. The cat is neurologically normal.

27. Palpate the muscles and bones, and flex and extend the joints.

27. The musculoskeletal system is normal.

28. Palpate the neck.

28. No abnormalities.

Go to Section C

Section C:

Which diagnostic procedures would you perform? *(Choose only the procedures you believe relevant to managing the case at this point.)*

29. Collect blood for a complete blood count.

29. The complete blood count results show the following:
PCV = 42%
Hb = 18.2 g/dl
RBC = 11.5 million/mm^3

MCV = 42 fl
MCHC = 33 g/dl
MCH = 15 pg
WBC = 10,800/mm^3
Segs = 7800/mm^3
Bands = 0/mm^3
Lymphocytes = 1800/mm^3
Monocytes = 600/mm^3
Eosinophils = 600/mm^3
Basophils = 0/mm^3
Platelets = 320,000/mm^3
Total protein = 6.2 g/dl

30. Collect blood for a serum glucose concentration.

30. Glucose = 185 mg/dl

31. Collect blood for a serum BUN and creatinine determination.

31. BUN = 66 mg/dl
Creatinine = 3.0 mg/dl

32. Collect blood for serum liver enzyme measurement.

32. ALT = 360 IU/L
GGT = 10 IU/L
SAP = 365 IU/L

33. Collect blood for calcium and phosphorus determination.

33. Calcium = 9.6 mg/dl
Phosphorus = 3.6 mg/dl

34. Collect blood for serum cholesterol measurement.

34. Cholesterol = 124 mg/dl

35. Collect blood for serum bilirubin measurement.

35. Bilirubin = 4.6 mg/dl
Direct bilirubin = 2.9 mg/dl
Indirect bilirubin = 1.7 mg/dl

36. Collect blood for a serum thyroid hormone concentration.

36. Serum thyroxine = 2.0 μg/dl

37. Collect urine for a urinalysis.

37. The urine was collected by free catch.
Color = dark yellow
Character = clear
Specific gravity = 1.058
pH = 6.5
Protein = negative
Glucose = negative
Ketones = negative
Bilirubin = 4+
Urobilinogen = negative
Blood = 2+
WBC = 1-3/hpf
RBC = 5-10/hpf
Epithelial cells/hpf = occasionally
Bacteria = negative
Casts = negative
Crystals = negative
Sperm = negative
Fat = negative

38. Collect blood for a feline leukemia virus test.

38. Negative.

39. Collect blood for a feline immunodeficiency virus test.

39. Negative.

40. Collect stool for fecal flotation.

40. Negative.

41. Obtain chest radiographs.

41. Normal.

42. Obtain abdominal radiographs.

42. Normal except for diffuse hepatomegaly.

43. Measure systolic and diastolic blood pressures.

43. Systolic blood pressure = 145 mm Hg; diastolic blood pressure = 85 mm Hg.

44. Perform an upper gastrointestinal study with barium.

44. Normal.

45. Collect blood for serum amylase and lipase determination.

45. Amylase = 200 IU/L
Lipase = 100 IU/L

Go to Section D

Section D:

Considering the information you have gained so far, what further diagnostic tests would you like to perform? *(Choose only the tests you believe relevant to managing the case at this point.)*

46. Collect blood for feline infectious peritonitis serology.

46. 1:100.

47. Collect fasting and postprandial blood samples for serum bile acid analysis.

47. Fasting serum bile acids = 165 mmol/L; postprandial serum bile acids = 200 mmol/L.

48. Perform a 24-hour creatinine clearance.

48. 2.8 ml/minute/kg.

49. Perform a funduscopic examination.

49. Normal.

50. Collect blood before and after administration of ACTH for serum cortisol analysis.

50. Pre-ACTH cortisol = 2.8 µg/dl; post-ACTH cortisol = 14.2 µg/dl.

51. Ultrasound the abdomen.

51. The liver is diffusely enlarged and more echogenic than usual. No masses are noted. Other abdominal organs are normal.

52. Collect blood for coagulation tests.

52. Prothrombin time = 8 seconds (normal = 6-10 seconds); Activated partial thromboplastin time = 10 seconds (normal = 12-18 seconds); Activated clotting time = 90 seconds (normal = 60-120 seconds); Platelet count = 320,000/mm^3.

53. Collect blood for *Toxoplasma* serology.

53. IgG = 1:4; IgM = 1:4.

54. Anesthetize the cat for a liver biopsy.

54. Biopsies pending.

55. Anesthetize the cat for endoscopic examination and gastrointestinal biopsies.

55. No abnormal findings; biopsies show a normal stomach mucosa and mild lymphoplasmacytic infiltrates in the mucosa of the duodenum.

56. Anesthetize the cat for renal biopsy.

56. Normal.

Go to Section E

Section E:

Which course of action would you take? *(Choose only one.)*

57. Prescribe methimazole and schedule a recheck examination in 2 weeks.

57. End of problem.

58. Prescribe metronidazole and prednisone at immunosuppressive doses and schedule a recheck examination in 1 week.

58. End of problem.

59. Prescribe amoxicillin and schedule a recheck examination in 2 weeks.

59. End of problem.

60. Initiate chemotherapy for lymphoma and schedule a recheck examination in 1 week.

60. End of problem.

61. Prescribe insulin therapy and recheck the cat in 1 week.

61. End of problem.

62. Advise the owners of the poor prognosis and recommend euthanasia.

62. End of problem.

63. Place an enteral feeding tube and provide nutritional requirements for the cat until the biopsy results are received.

63. End of problem.

END OF PROBLEM

Opening Scene:

The owner of a 5-year-old neutered male St. Bernard-Great Dane cross presents the dog to you with a complaint that the dog has acutely begun to vomit over the last hour. The dog has retched eight to 10 times and has been salivating profusely. He seems very uncomfortable and will not lie down. He lives in the western United States and has not traveled. He is up to date on his vaccinations, including distemper/parvovirus and rabies and is on monthly heartworm preventative.

Go to Section A

Section A:

What questions would you like to ask the owner? (*Choose only the questions you believe relevant to managing the case at this point.*)

1. Has he had any previous illnesses, injuries, or surgeries?

1. "He was neutered at 6 months of age."

2. Has there been any change in his thirst or urinary habits?

2. "No changes."

3. Is he currently on any medications?

3. "No."

4. What diet does he normally eat and about how much does he consume in a day?

4. "He eats a premium dry dog food, free choice. I couldn't really tell you how much he eats."

5. Is your dog weak or has he ever collapsed?

5. "Not usually, but he seems weak now."

6. What does the vomitus look like?

6. "Nothing is coming up. He retches and then it's like he has the dry heaves."

7. Has he had any diarrhea?

7. "No."

8. Has he been coughing or sneezing?

8. "No."

9. Has he been tested or treated for intestinal parasites?

9. "No."

10. Is there any possibility of toxin exposure?

10. "No."

11. Has he been fed table scraps or could he have gotten into the garbage?

11. "Sometimes we give him soup bones but none recently. He can't get into the garbage."

12. Has your dog had any changes in mental attitude or personality?

12. "No. "

13. Do you have any other pets?

13. "Yes, we have a cat but she's fine."

14. Has your dog ever had a seizure?

14. "Not that we've seen."

Section B:

Which physical examination procedures would you perform at this time? *(Choose only the procedures you believe relevant to managing the case at this point.)*

15. Measure the body weight.

15. 62.2 kg.

16. Measure the rectal body temperature.

16. 38.9°C.

17. Take the pulse and heart rate.

17. The heart rate is 192 beats per minute; the pulse is weak and thready.

18. Measure the respiratory rate and note the character of respirations.

18. The respiratory rate is 48 per minute.

19. Auscultate the lungs.

19. Lung sounds are normal.

20. Auscultate the heart.

20. Heart sounds are normal.

21. Examine the oral cavity.

21. The oral cavity is normal; mucous membranes are pale pink; capillary refill time is 2 seconds.

22. Palpate the peripheral lymph nodes.

22. Normal.

23. Palpate the abdomen.

23. The abdomen is distended and the dog resents palpation. The distension is primarily in the cranial abdomen just behind the ribs.

24. Examine the skin.

24. Normal.

25. Examine the ears, eyes, and nose.

25. No abnormalities.

26. Examine the neck and throat area.

26. Normal.

27. Assess cranial nerves, mental status, postural and spinal reflexes, gait and proprioception.

27. The dog is neurologically normal.

28. Palpate the muscles and bones, and flex and extend the joints.

28. The musculoskeletal system is normal.

Go to Section C

Section C:

Which diagnostic procedures would you perform? *(Choose only the procedures you believe relevant to managing the case at this point.)*

29. Collect blood for a complete blood count.

29. The complete blood count results show the following:
PCV = 48%
Hb = 12.2 g/dl
RBC = 8.5 million/mm^3
MCV = 68 fl

MCHC = 32 g/dl
MCH = 23 pg
WBC = 19,800/mm^3
Segs = 16,800/mm^3
Bands = 800/mm^3
Lymphocytes = 1200/mm^3
Monocytes = 400/mm^3
Eosinophils = 600/mm^3
Basophils = 0/mm^3
Platelets = 345,000/mm^3
Total protein = 7.0 g/dl

30. Collect blood for a serum BUN and creatinine.

30. BUN = 58 mg/dl
Creatinine = 2.6 mg/dl

31. Collect blood for serum liver enzyme analysis.

31. ALT = 260 IU/L
GGT = 1 IU/L
SAP = 65 IU/L

32. Collect blood for serum total protein and albumin measurement.

32. Albumin = 4.3 g/dl
Total protein = 7.0 g/dl

33. Collect blood for serum calcium and phosphorus measurement.

33. Calcium = 10.6 mg/dl
Phosphorus = 5.6 mg/dl

34. Collect blood for serum amylase and lipase determination.

34. Amylase (Harleco U) = 250
Lipase = 100

35. Collect blood for serum electrolyte quantitation.

35. Sodium = 145 mEq/L
Potassium = 2.4 mEq/L
Chloride = 108 mEq/L

36. Collect blood for serum blood glucose measurement.

36. Glucose = 105 mg/dl

37. Collect blood for serum cholesterol measurement.

37. Cholesterol = 100 mg/dl

38. Collect blood for serum bilirubin determination.

38. Total bilirubin = 0.1 mg/dl

39. Collect urine for a complete urinalysis.

39. The urine sample was collected by a catheter.
Color = yellow
Character = clear
Specific gravity = 1.047
pH = 6.5
Protein = negative
Glucose = negative
Ketones = negative
Bilirubin = 1+
Urobilinogen = negative
Blood = negative
WBC = 0-1/hpf
RBC = 3-5/hpf
Epithelial cells/hpf = occasionally
Bacteria = negative
Casts = negative

40. Collect stool for fecal flotation.

40. Negative.

41. Obtain chest radiographs.

41. Normal.

42. Obtain abdominal radiographs.

42. The stomach is gas-filled and distended. Compartmentalization of the stomach is evident with pyloric displacement dorsally and to the left.

43. Attempt to pass an orogastric tube.

43. The orogastric tube cannot be passed into the stomach. Decompression is not achieved.

44. Perform an electrocardiogram.

44. Sinus tachycardia.

Go to Section D

Section D:

Considering the information you have gained so far, what further diagnostic tests would you like to perform? *(Choose only the tests you believe relevant to managing the case at this point.)*

45. Collect blood for fasting and postprandial serum bile acids determination.

45. Fasting serum bile acids = 5 mmol/L; postprandial serum bile acids = 6 mmol/L.

46. Collect blood samples before and 1 and 2 hours after administering a high fat meal, and measure plasma turbidity.

46. Positive for lipemia at 1 and 2 hours postprandially.

47. Administer barium sulfate and perform an upper gastrointestinal radiographic series.

47. The barium does not pass into the stomach but stays in the esophagus.

48. Anesthetize the dog and perform intestinal biopsies by endoscopy.

48. The endoscope could not be passed into the stomach or small intestine; procedure aborted.

49. Perform an echocardiogram.

49. No abnormal findings.

50. Collect blood for trypsinlike immunoreactivity assay.

50. Results pending.

51. Use a 16 gauge needle to trocarize the dog in the right cranial abdomen.

51. The stomach is decompressed and the dog's cardiovascular status improves.

52. Perform a ventral midline abdominal paracentesis for the purpose of collecting peritoneal fluid.

52. No fluid is obtained.

53. Perform a barium esophagram.

53. Normal esophageal motility and shape.

54. Ultrasound the abdomen.

54. The procedure could not be performed adequately due to the large amount of gastric gas.

55. Collect blood pre- and post-ACTH administration for serum cortisol determination.

55. Pre-ACTH cortisol = 8 µg/dl; post-ACTH cortisol = 24.4 µg/dl.

56. Perform an ultrasound-guided liver biopsy.

56. Results pending.

Go to Section E

Section E:

Which course of action would you take? *(Choose only one.)*

57. Treat the dog symptomatically with intravenous fluids, antibiotics, and antiemetics and administer nothing per os.

57. End of problem.

58. Administer mineral oil by orogastric tube to stimulate gastrointestinal motility.

58. End of problem.

59. Administer atropine and 2-PAM and provide supportive care.

59. End of problem.

60. Administer intravenous fluids and glucocorticoids and perform abdominal surgery.

60. End of problem.

61. Refer the dog to a specialist for further workup.

61. End of problem.

62. Prescribe a protein-restricted diet and give the owners a poor prognosis.

62. End of problem.

END OF PROBLEM

Opening Scene:

The owner of a 3-year-old spayed female domestic shorthaired cat presents her cat to you with a complaint that the cat has been urinating outside the litter box for the past 4 weeks. She urinates more frequently than normal and the urine is sometimes red. The cat goes outdoors during the day but usually sleeps indoors at night. She is current on her vaccinations, including rabies.

Go to Section A

Section A:

What questions would you like to ask the owner? *(Choose only the questions you believe relevant to managing the case at this point.)*

1. Does your cat seem to be in pain when she urinates?

1. "Yes, she cries sometimes when she urinates."

2. How is your cat's appetite?

2. "Her appetite is fine."

3. Do you have other pets? If so, are any of them ill?

3. "Yes, we have two other cats, but they're fine."

4. Is there a possibility of an injury or traumatic incident?

4. "Not that I know of."

5. Has she had any previous illnesses, injuries, or surgeries?

5. "She has recurrently had problems like this but usually it goes away in a few days. Our vet usually gives us pink antibiotic drops for it. The only surgery she's had was her spay at 7 months of age."

6. What do you normally feed your cat?

6. "She eats free choice dry adult cat food."

7. Has there been any nasal or ocular discharge?

7. "No."

8. Have you found blood anywhere other than in her urine?

8. "Not that I've seen."

9. Has there been any change in your cat's drinking habits?

9. "She does seem to drink a little more than usual."

10. Does your cat appear to be lame?

10. "No."

11. Has your cat collapsed or had any seizures?

11. "Not that I have seen."

12. Has your cat had any changes in mental attitude or personality?

12. "She seems a little grouchy."

13. Has your cat been vomiting or had any diarrhea?

13. "No."

Section B:

Which physical examination procedures would you perform at this time? *(Choose only the procedures you believe relevant to managing the case at this point.)*

14. Measure the body weight.

14. 4.8 kg.

15. Measure the rectal body temperature.

15. 38.3°C.

16. Take the pulse and heart rate.

16. The heart rate is 144 beats per minute; the pulse is strong and regular.

17. Measure the respiratory rate and note the character of respirations.

17. The respiratory rate is 16 per minute.

18. Auscultate the lungs.

18. Lung sounds are normal.

19. Auscultate the heart.

19. Heart sounds are normal.

20. Examine the oral cavity.

20. Mild dental tartar; mucous membranes are pink; capillary refill time is 1 second.

21. Palpate the peripheral lymph nodes.

21. Normal.

22. Palpate the abdomen.

22. Normal except that the cat resents palpation of the caudal abdomen.

23. Examine the skin.

23. Normal.

24. Examine the ears, eyes, and nose.

24. No abnormalities with the ears, eyes, or nose.

25. Assess the hydration status.

25. Normal.

26. Assess cranial nerves, mental status, postural and spinal reflexes, gait and proprioception.

26. The cat is neurologically normal.

27. Palpate the muscles and bones, and flex and extend the joints.

27. The musculoskeletal system is normal.

28. Palpate the neck.

28. Normal.

Go to Section C

Section C:

Which diagnostic procedures would you perform? *(Choose only the procedures you believe relevant to managing the case at this point.)*

29. Collect blood for a complete blood count.

29. The complete blood count results show the following:
PCV = 42%
Hb = 18.2 g/dl
RBC = 11.5 million/mm^3

MCV = 42 fl
MCHC = 33 g/dl
MCH = 15 pg
WBC = 14,800/mm^3
Segs = 13,300/mm^3
Bands = 0/mm^3
Lymphocytes = 1200/mm^3
Monocytes = 100/mm^3
Eosinophils = 200/mm^3
Basophils = 0/mm^3
Platelets = 285,000/mm^3
Total protein = 6.5 g/dl

30. Collect blood for a serum BUN and creatinine determinations.

30. BUN = 16 mg/dl
Creatinine = 1.0 mg/dl

31. Collect blood for serum glucose measurement.

31. Glucose = 108 mg/dl

32. Collect blood for serum electrolyte measurement.

32. Sodium = 145 mEq/L
Potassium = 4.4 mEq/L
Chloride = 112 mEq/L

33. Collect blood for serum calcium and phosphorus measurement.

33. Calcium = 9.6 mg/dl
Phosphorus = 3.6 mg/dl

34. Collect blood for serum liver enzyme analysis.

34. ALT = 60 IU/L
GGT = 1 IU/L
SAP = 65 IU/L

35. Collect blood for serum bilirubin measurement.

35. Total bilirubin = 0.1 mg/dl

36. Collect urine for a urinalysis.

36. The urine was collected by cystocentesis.
Color = yellow
Character = clear
Specific gravity = 1.058
pH = 6.5
Protein = negative
Glucose = negative
Ketones = negative
Bilirubin = negative
Urobilinogen = negative
Blood = negative
WBC = 1-3/hpf
RBC = 20-30/hpf
Epithelial cells/hpf = occasionally
Bacteria = negative
Casts = negative
Crystals = 1+struvite
Sperm = negative
Fat = negative

37. Collect a urine sample for aerobic culture and antibiotic sensitivity.

37. No growth.

38. Collect blood for a feline leukemia virus test.

38. Negative.

39. Collect blood for a feline immunodeficiency virus test.

39. Negative.

40. Collect blood for a coagulation profile.

40. Activated partial thromboplastin time = 14 seconds (normal = 12-18 seconds); Prothrombin time = 8 seconds (normal = 6-10 seconds); Activated clotting time = 90 seconds (normal = 60-120 seconds); Platelet count = 289,000/ mm^3.

41. Obtain chest radiographs.

41. Normal.

42. Obtain abdominal radiographs.

42. Radiodense disc-shaped stone present in the urinary bladder; no other abnormalities.

Go to Section D

Section D:

Considering the information you have gained so far, what further diagnostic tests would you like to perform? (*Choose only the tests you believe relevant to managing the case at this point.*)

43. Perform a complete ophthalmological examination.

43. Normal.

44. Ultrasound the abdomen.

44. Solitary hyperechoic object consistent with a cystic calculi within the urinary bladder; other abdominal organs normal.

45. Perform a double contrast cystourethrogram.

45. The urinary bladder wall is thickened in the cranioventral area; 4 cm diameter filling defect in the contrast puddle within the urinary bladder; normal urethra.

46. Pass a urinary catheter to determine the patency of the lower urinary tract.

46. Urinary catheter passes easily into the bladder.

47. Collect blood for feline infectious peritonitis virus serology.

47. 1:100.

48. Collect blood for *Toxoplasma* serology.

48. IgG = 1:32; IgM = 1:16.

49. Collect blood for thyroid hormone analysis.

49. T$_4$ = 2.6 µg/dl.

50. Administer human chorionic gonadotropin (HCG) and measure plasma progesterone concentrations.

50. Pending.

51. Anesthetize the cat and perform an ultrasound-guided renal biopsy.

51. Normal renal tissue.

Section E:

Which course of action would you take? *(Choose only one.)*

52. Prescribe prednisone at an antiinflammatory dose to be tapered over the next 3 months to alternate day therapy.

    52. End of problem.

53. Prescribe diazepam and institute methods of behavioral modification.

    53. End of problem.

54. Prescribe progestogens and schedule a recheck examination in 2 weeks.

    54. End of problem.

55. Perform a cystotomy for stone removal and send the cat home on a low magnesium, urinary acidifying diet.

    55. End of problem.

56. Prescribe phenylpropanolamine and schedule a recheck examination in 2 weeks.

    56. End of problem.

57. Prescribe amoxicillin and schedule a recheck examination in 1 week.

    57. End of problem.

END OF PROBLEM

Opening Scene:

The owners of a 9-year-old intact female Miniature schnauzer present her to you with a history of anorexia and vomiting of 2 day's duration. Her appetite was decreased for 2 days before that and now she completely refuses food, even table scraps. She had all her vaccinations, including rabies 3 months ago. She is primarily an indoor dog and has access to a fenced-in backyard.

Go to Section A

Section A:

What questions would you like to ask the owner? *(Choose only the questions you believe relevant to managing the case at this point.)*

1. How many times has she vomited?

2. What does the vomitus look like?

3. What does she usually eat?

4. Is there a possibility of an injury or traumatic incident?

5. Has she had any previous illnesses, injuries, or surgeries?

6. Had she gotten into the garbage or had you given her table scraps before her getting sick?

7. Has she been around any strange or sick dogs?

8. Does your dog have any nasal or ocular discharge?

9. Has there been a change in her drinking or urinating habits?

10. Does your dog seem to be generally weak or depressed?

11. When was her last heat?

12. Has your dog collapsed or had any seizures?

13. Has she been coughing or sneezing?

14. Does she have diarrhea?

---

1. "She has vomited three times, twice yesterday and once today."

2. "It's just a yellowish foam."

3. "She normally eats a commercial canned dog food, a half a can twice a day."

4. "Not that I know of."

5. "No, she's always been healthy."

6. "No."

7. "No."

8. "Just a drop of clear fluid now and then."

9. "She has been drinking more than usual over the last week, and her urine is really light in color."

10. "She is very depressed and isn't interested in anything. She walks very slowly and seems to shake when she stands for a period of time."

11. "I think it was about 1½ to 2 months ago."

12. "Not that I have seen."

13. "No."

14. "She really hasn't passed any stool in 2 days, but before that it was normal."

Section B:

Which physical examination procedures would you perform at this time? *(Choose only the procedures you believe relevant to managing the case at this point.)*

15. Measure the body weight.

15. 17 kg.

16. Measure the rectal body temperature.

16. 40.3°C.

17. Take the pulse and heart rate.

17. The heart rate is 180 beats per minute; the pulse is strong and regular.

18. Measure the respiratory rate and note the character of respirations.

18. The respiratory rate is 48 per minute and normal.

19. Auscultate the lungs.

19. Lung sounds are normal.

20. Auscultate the heart.

20. Heart sounds are normal.

21. Examine the oral cavity.

21. The oral cavity is normal; mucous membranes are pink; capillary refill time is 2 seconds.

22. Assess the hydration status.

22. Skin turgor is decreased and the mucous membranes are tacky. Estimated 5% dehydration.

23. Palpate the peripheral lymph nodes.

23. Normal.

24. Palpate the abdomen.

24. A tubular mass is palpated in the ventral middle to caudal abdomen.

25. Examine the skin.

25. Normal.

26. Examine the ears, eyes, and nose.

26. No abnormalities.

27. Check for a vaginal discharge.

27. A mucopurulent vaginal discharge is matted around the vulva.

28. Assess cranial nerves, mental status, postural and spinal reflexes, gait and proprioception.

28. The dog is neurologically normal.

29. Palpate the muscles and bones, and flex and extend the joints.

29. The musculoskeletal system is normal.

Section C:

Which diagnostic procedures would you perform? *(Choose only the procedures you believe relevant to managing the case at this point.)*

30. Collect blood for a complete blood count.

30. The complete blood count results show the following:
PCV = 48%
Hb = 15.9 g/dl
RBC = 7.9 million/mm^3
MCV = 62 fl
MCHC = 32 g/dl
MCH = 23 pg
WBC = 41,800/mm^3
Segs = 35,500/mm^3
Bands = 4200/mm^3
Lymphocytes = 400/mm^3
Monocytes = 1700/mm^3
Eosinophils = 0/mm^3
Basophils = 0/mm^3
Platelets = 345,000/mm^3
Total protein = 7.8 g/dl

31. Collect blood for a serum glucose determination.

31. Glucose = 95 mg/dl

32. Collect blood for a serum BUN and creatinine measurement.

32. BUN = 16 mg/dl
Creatinine = 1.0 mg/dl

33. Collect blood for serum liver enzyme and bilirubin analysis.

33. ALT = 60 IU/L
GGT = 1 IU/L
SAP = 365 IU/L
Total bilirubin = 0.1 mg/dl

34. Collect blood for serum electrolyte measurement.

34. Sodium = 145 mEq/L
Potassium = 4.4 mEq/L
Chloride = 112 mEq/L

35. Collect blood for serum calcium and phosphorus determination.

35. Calcium = 9.6 mg/dl
Phosphorus = 3.6 mg/dl

36. Collect blood for serum cholesterol measurement.

36. Cholesterol = 100 mg/dl

37. Collect urine for a urinalysis.

37. The urine was collected by a catheter.
Color = yellow
Character = clear
Specific gravity = 1.038
pH = 6.5
Protein = negative
Glucose = negative
Ketones = negative
Bilirubin = negative
Urobilinogen = negative
Blood = negative
WBC = 1-3/hpf

RBC = 3-5/hpf
Epithelial cells/hpf = occasionally
Bacteria = negative
Casts = negative
Crystals = 1+struvite
Sperm = negative
Fat = negative

38. Obtain chest radiographs.

38. Normal.

39. Obtain abdominal radiographs.

39. A soft tissue density tubular mass is present in the ventral abdomen on the lateral view. On the ventrodorsal view, tubular masses are visible on both sides of the abdomen. The intestines are displaced craniodorsally. No other abnormalities are detected.

40. Perform an electrocardiogram.

40. Normal sinus rhythm.

41. Obtain feces for fecal flotation.

41. Negative.

42. Collect blood for serum amylase and lipase determination.

42. Amylase = 250 IU/L
Lipase = 100 IU/L

43. Perform an abdominocentesis to collect a sample of abdominal fluid.

43. No fluid obtained.

44. Collect a vaginal discharge sample for cytology.

44. Packed fields of degenerate neutrophils with intracellular rods.

45. Collect blood for aerobic and anaerobic bacterial cultures.

45. No growth.

46. Collect a urine sample for aerobic bacterial culture and antibiotic sensitivity.

46. No growth.

Go to Section D

Section D:

Considering the information you have gained so far, what further diagnostic tests would you like to perform?
(Choose only the tests you believe relevant to managing the case at this point.)

47. Collect blood for an ethylene glycol test.

47. Negative.

48. Collect blood before and after administering ACTH for plasma cortisol analysis.

48. Pre-ACTH cortisol = 4.5 µg/dl; post-ACTH cortisol = 21.3 µg/dl.

49. Collect vaginal discharge for aerobic bacterial culture and antibiotic sensitivity.

49. Heavy growth of *E.coli, Staphylococcus aureus,* and *Streptococcus fecalis* sensitive to multiple antibiotics.

50. Place an indwelling urinary catheter to monitor urine output.

50. Urine output = 65 ml/kg/day.

51. Perform an endogenous creatinine clearance test.

52. Perform a barium upper gastrointestinal radiographic series.

53. Perform an echocardiogram.

54. Anesthetize the dog for collection of bone marrow.

55. Ultrasound the abdomen.

56. Perform a water deprivation test.

51. 2.4 ml/kg/minute.

52. Normal.

53. Normal cardiac architecture and function.

54. Granulocytic hyperplasia.

55. Tubular anechoic mass consistent with the uterus is identified. No other abnormalities.

56. The dog looks more depressed and vomits three times within the first 2 hours.

Go to Section E

Section E:

Which course of action would you take? *(Choose only one.)*

57. Stabilize the dog with intravenous fluids and antibiotics and prepare for abdominal surgery.

58. Prescribe cephalexin and schedule a recheck examination in 1 week.

59. Recommend euthanasia due to the poor prognosis for recovery.

60. Treat the dog with intravenous fluids and give it nothing per os.

61. Prescribe an antiinflammatory dose of prednisone to be tapered over the next 3 weeks.

62. Instruct the owners to give the dog 25% less water than it usually drinks and schedule a recheck examination in 1 week.

57. End of problem.

58. End of problem.

59. End of problem.

60. End of problem.

61. End of problem.

62. End of problem.

END OF PROBLEM

Opening Scene:

The owner of a 12-year-old intact male domestic shorthaired cat presents his cat to you at your mixed animal country practice with a problem of excessive salivation and odor in the mouth. This problem has been present for the last 2 or 3 weeks and continues to get worse. He is an outdoor cat primarily but he does come in daily to eat. He is not current on his vaccinations.

Go to Section A

Section A:

What questions would you like to ask the owner? (*Choose only the questions you believe relevant to managing the case at this point.*)

1. Is there any possibility of exposure to caustic chemicals or other toxins?

   1. "It's possible as he's outside most of the time."

2. Has he ever had this problem before?

   2. "No."

3. Do you have other animals, and if so, are they well?

   3. "No, he's our only pet."

4. Has he ever had his teeth cleaned?

   4. "No."

5. Has he had any previous illnesses, injuries, or surgeries?

   5. "No."

6. How is his appetite and what is he normally fed?

   6. "He usually eats generic dry cat food but now he will only eat canned food, about a can a day."

7. Has there been any ocular or nasal discharge?

   7. "No."

8. Has he seemed less playful or active in the recent past?

   8. "No, he seems fine."

9. Has there been any change in your cat's thirst or urination habits?

   9. "No changes."

10. Has your cat vomited or had diarrhea recently?

    10. "No."

11. Has your cat collapsed or had any seizures?

    11. "Not that I have seen."

12. Has your cat had any changes in mental attitude or personality?

    12. "No."

13. When was your cat vaccinated last?

    13. "Three years ago."

Section B:

Which physical examination procedures would you perform at this time? (*Choose only the procedures you believe relevant to managing the case at this point.*)

14.	Measure the body weight.	14.	5.3 kg.
15.	Measure the rectal body temperature.	15.	38.3°C.
16.	Take the pulse and heart rate.	16.	The heart rate is 200 beats per minute; the pulse is strong and regular.
17.	Measure the respiratory rate and note the character of respirations.	17.	The respiratory rate is 16 per minute.
18.	Auscultate the lungs.	18.	Lung sounds are normal.
19.	Auscultate the heart.	19.	Heart sounds are normal.
20.	Examine the oral cavity.	20.	Mild dental tartar; mucous membranes are pale pink; capillary refill time is 1 second. A 2 by 3 cm ulcerated, proliferative mass is present in the left caudal pharynx.
21.	Palpate the peripheral lymph nodes.	21.	Submandibular lymph nodes are large and firm.
22.	Palpate the abdomen.	22.	Normal.
23.	Examine the skin.	23.	Hair coat is unkempt.
24.	Examine the ears, eyes, and nose.	24.	No abnormalities.
25.	Assess the hydration status.	25.	Hydration is normal.
26.	Assess cranial nerves, mental status, postural and spinal reflexes, gait and proprioception.	26.	Normal.
27.	Palpate the muscles and bones, and flex and extend the joints.	27.	Normal.
28.	Perform a funduscopic examination.	28.	The funduscopic exam is normal, except for old chorioretinitis scars.

Section C:

Which diagnostic procedures would you perform? *(Choose only the procedures you believe relevant to managing the case at this point.)*

29. Collect blood for a complete blood count.

29. The complete blood count results show the following:
PCV = 42%
Hb = 18.2 g/dl
RBC = 11.5 million/mm³
MCV = 42 fl
MCHC = 33 g/dl
MCH = 15 pg
WBC = 14,800/mm³
Segs = 11,800/mm³
Bands = 0/mm³
Lymphocytes = 1200/mm³
Monocytes = 1600/mm³
Eosinophils = 200/mm³
Basophils = 0/mm³
Platelets = 245,000/mm³
Total protein = 8.5 g/dl

30. Collect blood for a serum BUN and creatinine determination.

30. BUN = 16 mg/dl
Creatinine = 1.0 mg/dl

31. Collect blood for serum liver enzyme and bilirubin analysis.

31. ALT = 60 IU/L
GGT = 1 IU/L
SAP = 65 IU/L
Total bilirubin = 0.1 mg/dl

32. Collect blood for a serum glucose determination.

32. Glucose = 165 mg/dl.

33. Collect blood for serum cholesterol measurement.

33. Cholesterol = 100 mg/dl.

34. Collect blood for serum electrolyte measurement.

34. Sodium = 145 mEq/L
Potassium = 4.4 mEq/L
Chloride = 112 mEq/L

35. Collect blood for a feline leukemia virus test.

35. Negative.

36. Collect blood for a feline immunodeficiency virus test.

36. Negative.

37. Obtain chest radiographs.

37. Normal.

38. Obtain abdominal radiographs.

38. Normal.

39. Collect urine for a urinalysis.

39. The urine was collected by cystocentesis.
Color = yellow
Character = clear
Specific gravity = 1.058
pH = 6.5
Protein = negative

Glucose = negative
Ketones = negative
Bilirubin = negative
Urobilinogen = negative
Blood = negative
WBC = 1-3/hpf
RBC = 3-5/hpf
Epithelial cells/hpf = occasionally
Bacteria = negative
Casts = negative
Crystals = 1+struvite
Sperm = negative
Fat = negative

40. Collect a sample of saliva for cytological examination.

40. Predominate cell is a degenerate neutrophil; squamous epithelial cells also present; mixed populations of cocci and rods present in high numbers.

Go to Section D

Section D:

Considering the information you have gained so far, what further diagnostic tests would you like to perform? *(Choose only the tests you believe relevant to managing the case at this point.)*

41. Perform an endogenous creatinine clearance.

41. 3.0 ml/kg/minute.

42. Collect blood for protein electrophoresis.

42. Polyclonal gammopathy.

43. Collect urine for Bence-Jones protein determination.

43. Negative.

44. Anesthetize the cat for a complete oral examination and biopsies of the mouth.

44. Squamous cell carcinoma.

45. Collect blood for feline infectious peritonitis virus serology.

45. 1:100.

46. Collect blood for *Toxoplasma* serology.

46. IgG = 1:32; IgM = 1:16.

47. Collect aqueous humor by aqueocentesis.

47. Normal.

48. Collect samples by fine needle aspirate for the submandibular lymph nodes.

48. Reactive lymph node.

49. Collect blood for thyroid hormone analysis.

49. T_4 = 2.5 µg/dl.

Section E:

Which course of action would you take? *(Choose only one.)*

50. Prescribe prednisone at immunosuppressive dosages to be tapered over the next 3 months to alternate day therapy.

50. End of problem.

51. Perform a thorough teeth cleaning on the cat and prescribe amoxicillin for 2 weeks.

51. End of problem.

52. Prescribe a high dose of clindamycin for 21 days.

52. End of problem.

53. Refer the cat to a specialist for further diagnostics and treatment.

53. End of problem.

54. Euthanize the cat and have the brain examined for rabies.

54. End of problem.

55. Prescribe chlorhexidine mouthwash for the owner to flush the cat's mouth.

55. End of problem.

END OF PROBLEM

Opening Scene:

The owners of a 9-month-old male Rottweiler present their dog to you with a history of left rear limb lameness. The dog has been lame off and on for the past 4 weeks. It began with the right hind leg and now affects the left hind leg. He is up to date on all his vaccinations, including rabies. He is primarily an indoor dog and has access to a fenced-in backyard. He lives in the midwestern United States.

Go to Section A

Section A:

What questions would you like to ask the owner? *(Choose only the questions you believe relevant to managing the case at this point.)*

1. Has he favored either of his front legs?

2. Is there any possibility of trauma?

3. What do you feed him and how much does he eat?

4. Is he on any dietary supplements?

5. Has he had any previous illnesses, injuries, or surgeries?

6. Is he receiving any medications?

7. Has he been around any strange or sick dogs?

8. Have you found any ticks on him?

9. Has he traveled with you anywhere?

10. Has he vomited or had diarrhea?

11. Has he been coughing or sneezing?

12. Has your dog collapsed or had any seizures?

13. Has your dog had any changes in mental attitude or personality?

14. Has there been any change in your dog's water consumption or urinary habits?

1. "Yes, he favored his right front leg for a day about a week ago."

2. "No, that's not possible."

3. "He eats a high protein dog food from a self feeder and a lot of it. Except lately, I haven't had to fill it as often."

4. "Yes, he's on a calcium/phosphorus supplement."

5. "No."

6. "No."

7. "No."

8. "Yeah, we pulled some ticks off of him about a month ago."

9. "No."

10. "Well, he has had a loose stool for the past week."

11. "No."

12. "Not that I have seen."

13. "He hasn't been as playful as usual. Usually he brings his toys to us constantly so we'll play with him, but he hasn't done that in the last week."

14. "No."

Section B:

Which physical examination procedures would you perform at this time? *(Choose only the procedures you believe relevant to managing the case at this point.)*

15. Measure the body weight.	15. 41 kg.
16. Measure the rectal body temperature.	16. 40.6°C.
17. Take the pulse and heart rate.	17. The heart rate is 120 beats per minute; the pulse is strong and regular.
18. Measure the respiratory rate and note the character of respirations.	18. The respiratory rate is 24 per minute and respirations are normal.
19. Auscultate the lungs.	19. Lung sounds are normal.
20. Auscultate the heart.	20. Heart sounds are normal.
21. Examine the oral cavity.	21. The oral cavity is normal; mucous membranes are pink; capillary refill time is 1 second.
22. Assess the hydration status.	22. Normal.
23. Palpate the peripheral lymph nodes.	23. Normal.
24. Palpate the abdomen.	24. No abnormalities detected.
25. Examine the skin.	25. Normal.
26. Examine the ears, eyes, and nose.	26. No abnormalities.
27. Examine the feet and pads.	27. Normal.
28. Assess cranial nerves, mental status, postural and spinal reflexes, gait and proprioception.	28. The dog is neurologically normal.
29. Palpate the muscles and bones, and flex and extend the joints.	29. Pain is elicited on manipulation of the stifles and on deep palpation of the distal femur. No other abnormalities detected.

Go to Section C

Section C:

Which diagnostic procedures would you perform? *(Choose only the procedures you believe relevant to managing the case at this point.)*

30. Collect blood for a complete blood count.	30. The complete blood count results show the following: PCV = 42% Hb = 15.2 g/dl RBC = 7.5 million/mm^3

MCV = 62 fl
MCHC = 32 g/dl
MCH = 23 pg
WBC = 21,200/mm^3
Segs = 17,600/mm^3
Bands = 0/mm^3
Lymphocytes = 2000/mm^3
Monocytes = 800/mm^3
Eosinophils = 800/mm^3
Basophils = 0/mm^3
Platelets = 245,000/mm^3
Total protein = 5.5 g/dl

31. Collect blood for a serum glucose determination.

31. Glucose = 105 mg/dl

32. Collect blood for serum calcium and phosphorus measurement.

32. Calcium = 12.6 mg/dl
Phosphorus = 9.6 mg/dl

33. Collect blood for serum alkaline phosphatase determination.

33. SAP = 365 IU/L.

34. Collect blood for BUN and creatinine measurement.

34. BUN = 16 mg/dl
Creatinine = 0.8 mg/dl

35. Collect blood for serum electrolyte determination.

35. Sodium = 134 mEq/L
Potassium = 2.4 mEq/L
Chloride = 92 mEq/L

36. Collect blood for a Knott's test.

36. Negative.

37. Collect urine for a urinalysis.

37. The urine was collected free catch.
Color = yellow
Character = clear
Specific gravity = 1.048
pH = 6.0
Protein = negative
Glucose = negative
Ketones = negative
Bilirubin = 2+
Urobilinogen = trace
Blood = negative
WBC = 1-3/hpf
RBC = 3-5/hpf
Epithelial cells/hpf = occasionally
Bacteria = negative
Casts = negative
Crystals = negative
Sperm = negative
Fat = negative

38. Obtain chest radiographs.

38. Normal.

39. Obtain abdominal radiographs.

39. Normal.

40. Radiograph the right and left femurs and stifles.	40. Generalized increased density in the diaphyseal portion of the medullary cavity of both femurs; stifles are radiographically normal.
41. Obtain feces for fecal flotation.	41. Negative.
42. Anesthetize the dog for arthrocentesis of the carpus, stifle, and tarsus for cytological examination.	42. Normal.
43. Radiograph the right and left humeri and shoulders.	43. Generalized increase in density of the diaphyseal portion of the medullary cavity of the humerus. Shoulders are radiographically normal.
44. Radiograph both carpi and tarsi.	44. Normal.
45. Collect blood for aerobic and anaerobic cultures.	45. No growth.
46. Radiograph the hip joints.	46. Normal.

Go to Section D

Section D:

Considering the information you have gained so far, what further diagnostic tests would you like to perform? *(Choose only the tests you believe relevant to managing the case at this point.)*

47. Collect blood for a Lyme's titer.	47. 1:32.
48. Collect blood for an antinuclear antibody test.	48. Negative.
49. Anesthetize the dog for arthrocentesis for aerobic and anaerobic bacterial culture and antibiotic sensitivity.	49. No growth.
50. Anesthetize the dog for bone biopsy.	50. Pending.
51. Anesthetize the dog for exploratory surgery of the stifle joints.	51. Scheduled.
52. Collect blood before and after a meal for serum bile acid determination.	52. Preprandial serum bile acids = 5 μmol/L; postprandial serum bile acids = 10 μmol/L.
53. Collect blood before and after administration of ACTH for plasma cortisol measurement.	53. Pre-ACTH cortisol = 6.6 μg/dl; post-ACTH cortisol = 14 μg/dl.
54. Perform lymph node aspiration biopsies.	54. Normal lymph node.
55. Collect blood for serum parathyroid hormone analysis.	55. Pending.

Section E:

Which course of action would you take? *(Choose only one.)*

56. Prescribe cephalexin for 3 weeks and schedule a recheck examination at that time.

    56. End of problem.

57. Administer a Lyme vaccine and schedule a recheck examination in 1 week.

    57. End of problem.

58. Administer prednisone at antiinflammatory doses for 3 weeks followed by a slow tapering of the dose over the next 3 weeks.

    58. End of problem.

59. Prescribe prednisone at immunosuppressive doses followed by a slow tapering of the dose over the next 3 months.

    59. End of problem.

60. Administer glycosaminoglycans by intramuscular injection and schedule a recheck examination in 1 week.

    60. End of problem.

61. Refer the dog to an orthopedic surgeon for total hip replacement.

    61. End of problem.

62. Send the dog home with instructions for cage rest and aspirin therapy as needed as well as a change in diet to adult maintenance without supplementation.

    62. End of problem.

END OF PROBLEM

Opening Scene:

The owner of a 2-year-old neutered male domestic shorthair cat presents the cat to you with a soft mass under his right front leg. This was first noticed yesterday and has grown considerably in the last 24 hours. He is an indoor and outdoor cat that lives on a farm in the midwestern United States. He is current on his vaccinations, including rabies.

Go to Section A

Section A:

What questions would you like to ask the owner? *(Choose only the questions you believe relevant to managing the case at this point.)*

1. Is there any possibility of injury or traumatic incident?

2. Does he ever fight with the neighborhood cats?

3. Do you have other pets?

4. Is he on any medications?

5. Has he had any previous illnesses, injuries, or surgeries?

6. Has he exhibited any difficulty breathing?

7. Has there been any ocular or nasal discharge?

8. Has he seemed less playful or active in the recent past?

9. Has there been any change in your cat's thirst or urination habits?

10. Has your cat vomited or had diarrhea recently?

11. Has your cat collapsed or had any seizures?

12. Has your cat had any changes in mental attitude or personality?

13. What do you normally feed your cat?

14. Is there a possibility of exposure to toxins?

1. "I don't know of any."

2. "Sometimes I hear the cats fighting, but I haven't heard anything recently."

3. "Yes, we have a dog. The two of them get along great."

4. "No."

5. "No, just his neuter at 6 months of age."

6. "No."

7. "No."

8. "He seems real quiet this morning."

9. "No changes."

10. "No."

11. "Not that I have seen."

12. "No."

13. "He eats a high quality commercial dry cat food free choice. He has been eating fine, but I don't think he ate much this morning."

14. "Anything is possible since he goes outdoors."

Go to Section B

Section B:

Which physical examination procedures would you perform at this time? *(Choose only the procedures you believe relevant to managing the case at this point.)*

15. Measure the rectal body temperature.

16. Take the pulse and heart rate.

17. Measure the respiratory rate and note the character of respirations.

18. Auscultate the lungs.

19. Auscultate the heart.

20. Examine the oral cavity.

21. Palpate the peripheral lymph nodes.

22. Palpate the abdomen.

23. Examine the skin.

24. Examine the ears, eyes, and nose.

25. Palpate the mass.

26. Assess cranial nerves, mental status, postural and spinal reflexes, gait and proprioception.

27. Palpate the muscles and bones, and flex and extend the joints.

28. Perform a funduscopic examination.

---

15. 37.9°C.

16. The heart rate is 200 beats per minute; the pulse is strong and regular.

17. The respiratory rate is 72 per minute and respirations are shallow.

18. Lung sounds are harsh.

19. Heart sounds are normal.

20. Mucous membranes are pale pink and moist; capillary refill time is 1 second.

21. Normal.

22. No abnormalities are noted on abdominal palpation.

23. Normal.

24. No abnormalities.

25. A soft, fluctuant mass that measures 6 by 8 cm is present in the subcutaneous tissues of the right axillary region.

26. Normal.

27. Normal.

28. The funduscopic exam reveals multifocal pinpoint retinal hemorrhages.

Go to Section C

Section C:

Which diagnostic procedures would you perform? *(Choose only the procedures you believe relevant to managing the case at this point.)*

29. Collect blood for a complete blood count.

---

29. The complete blood count results show the following:
PCV = 14%
Hb = 5.2 g/dl

RBC = 3.5 million/mm^3
MCV = 42 fl
MCHC = 33 g/dl
MCH = 15 pg
WBC = 24,600/mm^3
Segs = 23,400/mm^3
Bands = 0/mm^3
Lymphocytes = 800/mm^3
Monocytes = 200/mm^3
Eosinophils = 200/mm^3
Basophils = 0/mm^3
Platelets = 210,000/mm^3
Total protein = 5.5 g/dl

30. Collect blood for a serum BUN and creatinine measurement.

30. BUN = 11 mg/dl
Creatinine = 0.6 mg/dl

31. Collect blood for serum liver enzyme determination.

31. ALT = 126 IU/L
GGT = 1 IU/L
SAP = 65 IU/L
Total bilirubin = 0.2 mg/dl

32. Collect blood for serum glucose determination.

32. Glucose = 168 mg/dl.

33. Collect blood for serum electrolyte measurement.

33. Sodium = 145 mEq/L
Potassium = 3.4 mEq/L
Chloride = 112 mEq/L

34. Collect blood for serum calcium and phosphorus measurement.

34. Calcium = 9.6 mg/dl
Phosphorus = 3.6 mg/dl

35. Collect urine for a urinalysis.

35. The urine was collected free catch.
Color = dark yellow
Character = clear
Specific gravity = 1.058
pH = 6.5
Protein = negative
Glucose = negative
Ketones = negative
Bilirubin = negative
Urobilinogen = negative
Blood = 2+
WBC = 1-3/hpf
RBC = 20-30/hpf
Epithelial cells/hpf = occasionally
Bacteria = negative
Casts = negative
Crystals = negative
Sperm = negative
Fat = negative

36. Obtain radiographs of the mass.

36. Soft tissue density mass in the right axilla.

37. Obtain chest radiographs.

37. Patchy areas of alveolar disease throughout the lung fields. The heart is radiographically normal.

38. Perform a fine needle aspiration of the mass.

38. Approximately 3 ml of fluid obtained; cytology is consistent with hemorrhage.

39. Collect blood for a feline leukemia virus test.

39. Negative.

40. Collect blood for a feline immunodeficiency virus test.

40. Negative.

Go to Section D

Section D:

Considering the information you have gained so far, what further diagnostic tests would you like to perform? (*Choose only the tests you believe relevant to managing the case at this point.*)

41. Anesthetize the cat and perform a biopsy of the mass.

41. Pending.

42. Sedate the cat and lance and drain the mass.

42. The mass is lanced and sanguineous fluid drains from the opening.

43. Collect fasting and postprandial blood samples for serum bile acid determination.

43. Fasting serum bile acids = 2 μmol/L; postprandial serum bile acids = 5 μmol/L.

44. Collect blood for coagulation studies.

44. Prothrombin time = 32 seconds (normal = 6-10 seconds); Partial thromboplastin time = 25 seconds (normal = 12-18 seconds); Activated clotting time = 285 seconds (normal = 60-120 seconds); Platelet count = 210,000/mm^3.

45. Measure the cat's blood pressure.

45. 156/82 mm Hg.

46. Perform a thoracocentesis.

46. No fluid obtained.

47. Sedate the cat for a transoral tracheal wash to collect respiratory samples for cytology and bacterial culture.

47. Cytology consistent with hemorrhage; no bacteria seen.

48. Collect blood for a Coomb's test.

48. Negative.

Go to Section E

Section E:

Which course of action would you take? (*Choose only one.*)

49. Prescribe antibiotics and instruct the owner to hot pack the mass three times daily; recheck the cat in 1 week.

49. End of problem.

50. Recommend complete surgical excision of the mass.

50. End of problem.

51. Recommend euthanasia due to the poor prognosis.

51. End of problem.

52. Administer vitamin K1 by injection and administer a fresh whole blood transfusion.

52. End of problem.

53. Prescribe prednisone at immunosuppressive doses and schedule a recheck examination in 1 week.

53. End of problem.

END OF PROBLEM

Opening Scene:

The owner of a 12-year-old neutered male Brittany spaniel presents the dog to you with a complaint that the dog is weak and depressed. Also, he has had one fit. He is an indoor dog that has access to a fenced backyard. He lives in the midwestern United States and has not traveled. He is current on his vaccinations, including rabies, and is on monthly heartworm preventative.

Go to Section A

Section A:

What questions would you like to ask the owner? (*Choose only the questions you believe relevant to managing the case at this point.*)

1. Can you describe the fit?

2. What was he doing before the fit?

3. Why do you think your dog is weak?

4. What does he normally eat and how is his appetite?

5. Has he had any previous illnesses, injuries, or surgeries?

6. Has he been coughing or sneezing?

7. Does he vomit or have diarrhea?

8. Has there been any hair loss or other skin problems?

9. Has he lost any weight?

10. Is your dog on any medications other than heartworm preventative?

11. Does your dog favor any of his legs when he walks?

12. Has your dog had any changes in mental attitude or personality?

13. Is there any possibility of toxin exposure?

14. Could he have been injured recently?

---

1. "He got stiff and fell to one side. Then his neck arched backwards and he began paddling and salivating. It lasted about 45 seconds and at the end he urinated."

2. "He was just laying around and then got up to walk to his water dish."

3. "He seems to prefer to lay around. When he gets up, he moves slowly. If he stands for any length of time, he begins to tremble."

4. "He eats high quality dry food and his appetite seems good."

5. "Other than his neuter, he's had no surgeries or other problems for that matter."

6. "Not that I've noticed."

7. "No."

8. "No."

9. "He has lost a couple pounds."

10. "No."

11. "No."

12. "He just seems depressed and not interested in much."

13. "Nope."

14. "Not that we've seen."

Section B:

Which physical examination procedures would you perform at this time? *(Choose only the procedures you believe relevant to managing the case at this point.)*

15. Measure the body weight.

16. Measure the rectal body temperature.

17. Take the pulse and heart rate.

18. Measure the respiratory rate and note the character of respirations.

19. Auscultate the lungs.

20. Auscultate the heart.

21. Examine the oral cavity.

22. Palpate the peripheral lymph nodes.

23. Palpate the abdomen.

24. Examine the skin.

25. Examine the ears, eyes, and nose.

26. Examine the neck and throat area.

27. Assess cranial nerves, mental status, postural and spinal reflexes, gait and proprioception.

28. Palpate the muscles and bones, and flex and extend the joints.

15. 16 kg.

16. 37.9°C.

17. The heart rate is 108 beats per minute; the pulse is strong and regular.

18. The respiratory rate is 24 per minute.

19. Lung sounds are normal.

20. Heart sounds are normal.

21. The oral cavity is normal; mucous membranes are pink; capillary refill time is 1 second.

22. Normal.

23. Normal.

24. Normal.

25. No abnormalities.

26. Normal.

27. The dog is neurologically normal.

28. The musculoskeletal system is normal.

Go to Section C

Section C:

Which diagnostic procedures would you perform? *(Choose only the procedures you believe relevant to managing the case at this point.)*

29. Collect blood for a complete blood count.

29. The complete blood count results show the following:
PCV = 38%
Hb = 13.2 g/dl
RBC = 7.5 million/mm^3
MCV = 68 fl
MCHC = 32 g/dl
MCH = 23 pg

WBC = 11,800/mm^3
Segs = 9800/mm^3
Bands = 0/mm^3
Lymphocytes = 1200/mm^3
Monocytes = 600/mm^3
Eosinophils = 200/mm^3
Basophils = 0/mm^3
Platelets = 245,000/mm^3
Total protein = 6.5 g/dl

30. Collect blood for a serum BUN and creatinine.

30. BUN = 16 mg/dl
Creatinine = 1.4 mg/dl

31. Collect blood for liver enzyme analysis.

31. ALT = 260 IU/L
GGT = 1 IU/L
SAP = 65 IU/L

32. Collect blood for serum total protein and albumin measurement.

32. Albumin = 3.5 g/dl
Total protein = 6.5 g/dl

33. Collect blood for serum calcium and phosphorus measurement.

33. Calcium = 10.6 mg/dl
Phosphorus = 4.6 mg/dl

34. Collect blood for serum amylase and lipase determination.

34. Amylase = 250 IU/L
Lipase = 100 IU/L

35. Collect blood for serum electrolyte quantitation.

35. Sodium = 145 mEq/L
Potassium = 4.4 mEq/L
Chloride = 112 mEq/L

36. Collect blood for serum blood glucose measurement.

36. Glucose = 45 mg/dl.

37. Collect blood for serum cholesterol measurement.

37. Cholesterol = 100 mg/dl.

38. Collect blood for serum bilirubin determination.

38. Total bilirubin = 0.1 mg/dl.

39. Collect urine for a complete urinalysis.

39. The urine was collected by cystocentesis.
Color = yellow
Character = clear
Specific gravity = 1.037
pH = 6.5
Protein = negative
Glucose = negative
Ketones = negative
Bilirubin = 1+
Urobilinogen = negative
Blood = negative
WBC = 1-3/hpf
RBC = 3-5/hpf
Epithelial cells/hpf = occasionally
Bacteria = negative
Casts = negative
Crystals = 1+ calcium oxalate
Sperm = negative
Fat = negative

40. Radiograph the abdomen.	40. No abnormal findings.
41. Radiograph the chest.	41. No abnormal findings.
42. Anesthetize the dog for skull radiographs.	42. Normal.
43. Collect blood for lead analysis.	43. Blood lead < 0.04 ppm.
44. Perform a fundic examination.	44. Normal.

Go to Section D

Section D:

Considering the information you have gained so far, what further diagnostic tests would you like to perform? (*Choose only the tests you believe relevant to managing the case at this point.*)

45. Collect blood before and 2 hours after a meal for serum bile acid determination.	45. Preprandial bile acids = 5 mmol/L; postprandial bile acids = 6 mmol/L.
46. Collect blood for canine distemper titer.	46. Serum canine distemper titer = 1:2.
47. Anesthetize the dog for collection of cerebrospinal fluid.	47. Normal.
48. Refer the dog to a specialist for a computerized tomogram of the brain.	48. Normal.
49. Ultrasound the abdomen.	49. The liver has multifocal 1 cm areas of hypoechogenicity. No other abnormalities are noted.
50. Collect a fasting blood sample for paired serum glucose and insulin assays.	50. Fasting blood glucose = 39 mg/dl; blood insulin = 110 pmol/L (normal = 60-120 pmol/L).
51. Sedate the dog for hip radiographs.	51. No abnormal findings.
52. Collect blood for anaerobic and aerobic blood cultures and antibiotic sensitivity.	52. No growth.
53. Obtain an electrocardiogram.	53. Normal.
54. Obtain an echocardiogram.	54. Normal.
55. Collect blood pre- and post-ACTH administration for serum cortisol determination.	55. Pre-ACTH cortisol = 3.4 µg/dl; post-ACTH cortisol = 14.1 µg/dl.

Section E:

Which course of action would you take? *(Choose only one.)*

56. Prescribe oral prednisone at a dose of 1.0 mg/kg daily and recheck the serum chemistry panel.

    56. End of problem.

57. Administer intravenous 5% dextrose and schedule the dog for exploratory laparotomy.

    57. End of problem.

58. Recommend that a liver biopsy be done to determine the cause of the problem.

    58. End of problem.

59. Prescribe a high protein diet to be given in four daily feedings.

    59. End of problem.

60. Prescribe insulin therapy and schedule a recheck examination in 1 week.

    60. End of problem.

61. Prescribe phenobarbital and schedule a recheck examination in 2 weeks.

    61. End of problem.

END OF PROBLEM

PROBLEM 37

Opening Scene:

The owner of a 4-year-old spayed female domestic shorthaired cat presents her cat to you with a problem of diarrhea of 6 weeks duration. The cat's appetite is very good but she has lost about 1 kg of body weight. The cat is an indoor and outdoor cat. She is current on her vaccinations, including rabies.

Go to Section A

Section A:

What questions would you like to ask the owner? (*Choose only the questions you believe relevant to managing the case at this point.*)

1. Has she had any previous illnesses, injuries, or surgeries?

2. What is her diet and how much does she eat daily?

3. Is she on any medications?

4. Is there blood or mucus in the stool?

5. How frequently does she have a bowel movement?

6. Does she strain to defecate?

7. Has there been a change in her water consumption?

8. Has your cat been vomiting?

9. Do you have other animals?

10. Has she been treated for intestinal parasites?

11. Has your cat collapsed or had any seizures?

12. Has your cat had any changes in mental attitude or personality?

13. Does your cat have any skin disease?

1. "No, just her spay surgery."

2. "She eats a high quality dry cat food free choice and gets a few tablespoons of canned cat food twice a day. Her appetite is great."

3. "No."

4. "No."

5. "She goes about three times a day."

6. "No."

7. "She drinks a little more than usual."

8. "She has vomited three or four times in the past 6 weeks."

9. "Yes, we have a dog, too, but she's fine."

10. "Only when she was a kitten."

11. "Not that I have seen."

12. "Her attitude is great."

13. "No."

Section B:

Which physical examination procedures would you perform at this time? *(Choose only the procedures you believe relevant to managing the case at this point.)*

14. Measure the rectal body temperature.

14. 38.3°C.

15. Take the pulse and heart rate.

15. The heart rate is 144 beats per minute; the pulse is strong and regular.

16. Measure the respiratory rate and note the character of respirations.

16. The respiratory rate is 16 per minute.

17. Auscultate the lungs.

17. Lung sounds are normal.

18. Auscultate the heart.

18. Heart sounds are normal.

19. Examine the oral cavity.

19. Mild dental tartar; mucous membranes are pink; capillary refill time is 1 second.

20. Palpate the peripheral lymph nodes.

20. Normal.

21. Palpate the abdomen.

21. Normal except for thickened bowel loops.

22. Examine the skin.

22. Normal.

23. Examine the ears, eyes, and nose.

23. No abnormalities.

24. Assess the hydration status.

24. Normal.

25. Assess cranial nerves, mental status, postural and spinal reflexes, gait and proprioception.

25. The cat is neurologically normal.

26. Palpate the muscles and bones, and flex and extend the joints.

26. The musculoskeletal system is normal.

27. Palpate the neck.

27. No abnormalities.

Go to Section C

Section C:

Which diagnostic procedures would you perform? *(Choose only the procedures you believe relevant to managing the case at this point.)*

28. Collect blood for a complete blood count.

28. The complete blood count results show the following:
PCV = 42%
Hb = 18.2 g/dl
RBC = 11.5 million/mm^3
MCV = 42 fl
MCHC = 33 g/dl
MCH = 15 pg

WBC = 14,800/mm^3
Segs = 12,800/mm^3
Bands = 0/mm^3
Lymphocytes = 1800/mm^3
Monocytes = 1000/mm^3
Eosinophils = 1200/mm^3
Basophils = 0/mm^3
Platelets = 285,000/mm^3
Total protein = 6.5 g/dl

29. Collect blood for a serum glucose concentration.

29. Glucose = 145 mg/dl

30. Collect blood for a BUN and creatinine determination.

30. BUN = 20 mg/dl
Creatinine = 1.2 mg/dl

31. Collect blood for serum liver enzyme and bilirubin measurement.

31. ALT = 60 IU/L
GGT = 1 IU/L
SAP = 64 IU/L
Bilirubin = 0.1 mg/dl

32. Collect blood for calcium and phosphorus determination.

32. Calcium = 9.6 mg/dl
Phosphorus = 3.6 mg/dl

33. Collect blood for serum cholesterol measurement.

33. Cholesterol = 124 mg/dl.

34. Collect stool for fecal flotation.

34. Negative.

35. Collect blood for a serum thyroid hormone concentration.

35. Serum thyroxine = 2.0 μg/dl.

36. Collect urine for a urinalysis.

36. The urine was collected by cystocentesis.
Color = yellow
Character = clear
Specific gravity = 1.048
pH = 6.5
Protein = negative
Glucose = negative
Ketones = negative
Bilirubin = negative
Urobilinogen = negative
Blood = negative
WBC = 1-3/hpf
RBC = 3-5/hpf
Epithelial cells/hpf = occasionally
Bacteria = negative
Casts = negative
Crystals = negative
Sperm = negative
Fat = negative

37. Collect blood for a feline leukemia virus test.

37. Negative.

38. Collect blood for a feline immunodeficiency virus test.

38. Negative.

39. Collect stool to examine for the presence of fecal fat, starch, and trypsin.

39. Increased fecal fat; no starch seen; trypsin present.

40. Obtain chest radiographs.

40. Normal.

41. Obtain abdominal radiographs.

41. Normal.

42. Collect stool for aerobic and anaerobic bacterial culture and antibiotic sensitivity.

42. Heavy growth of *E. coli* sensitive to most antibiotics.

43. Administer barium and perform an upper gastrointestinal radiographic series.

43. Normal with the exception of diffusely thickened bowel walls.

44. Perform a fundic examination.

44. Normal.

Go to Section D

Section D:

Considering the information you have gained so far, what further diagnostic tests would you like to perform? *(Choose only the tests you believe relevant to managing the case at this point.)*

45. Perform a T_3 suppression test.

45. The serum $T_4 = 2.0$ µg/dl before administration of T_3; post-T_3 administration, the $T_4 = 0.5$ µg/dl (normal < 1.5 µg/dl).

46. Collect blood for a serum trypsinlike immuno-reactivity assay.

46. Normal.

47. Collect blood before and after ACTH administration for serum cortisol measurement.

47. Pre-ACTH cortisol = 3.9 µg/dl; post-ACTH cortisol = 6.3 µg/dl.

48. Perform a plasma turbidity test.

48. Normal.

49. Collect fasting and postprandial blood samples for serum bile acid analysis.

49. Fasting serum bile acids = 3 mmol/L; postprandial serum bile acids = 5 mmol/L.

50. Perform a barium enema.

50. Normal.

51. Collect blood for feline infectious peritonitis virus serology.

51. 1:100.

52. Collect blood for *Toxoplasma* serology.

52. IgG = 1:4; IgM = 1:4.

53. Anesthetize the cat for upper gastrointestinal endoscopy.

53. The stomach is grossly normal; duodenum is thickened, friable, and granular in appearance; biopsies reveal severe lymphoplasmacytic gastroenteritis.

54. Anesthetize the cat for colonoscopy.

54. No abnormal findings.

55. Ultrasound the abdomen.

55. Normal.

Section E:

Which course of action would you take? *(Choose only one.)*

56. Prescribe methimazole and schedule a recheck examination in 2 weeks.

56. End of problem.

57. Give the cat nothing per os for 24 hours and administer subcutaneous fluids to maintain hydration.

57. End of problem.

58. Prescribe amoxicillin and schedule a recheck examination in 2 weeks.

58. End of problem.

59. Prescribe enzyme replacement therapy to be added to the food and schedule a recheck examination in 2 weeks.

59. End of problem.

60. Prescribe prednisone at physiological doses and schedule a recheck examination in 2 weeks.

60. End of problem.

61. Treat the cat with fenbendazole and prescribe immunosuppressive doses of prednisone. Schedule a recheck examination in 2 weeks.

61. End of problem.

END OF PROBLEM

Opening Scene:

The owner of a 7-year-old neutered male Shar Pei complains to you that his dog is losing weight. His appetite seems decreased. He lives in the western United States and has not traveled. He has had all his vaccinations, including rabies, and is on monthly heartworm preventative.

Go to Section A

Section A:

What questions would you like to ask the owner? *(Choose only the questions you believe relevant to managing the case at this point.)*

1. Has he had any previous illnesses, injuries, or surgeries?

   1. "No."

2. Has there been any change in his thirst or urinary habits?

   2. "No."

3. Has he been coughing or sneezing?

   3. "No."

4. What does he normally eat and how much is he eating?

   4. "He eats a generic dry dog food, but he's consuming about half of his usual amount, maybe 1 cup per day."

5. Is your dog weak? Has he ever collapsed?

   5. "No."

6. Is your dog lame?

   6. "No."

7. Does he vomit or have diarrhea?

   7. "He vomits about twice a week and has a loose stool about half the time. It seems like for the past 2 months, he's just had a touchy stomach. The stool is light brown in color and soft. There is no blood or mucus in it."

8. Have you noticed any itching or other skin disease?

   8. "No."

9. Other than heartworm preventative, is your dog on any medications?

   9. "No."

10. Is there any possibility of toxin exposure? Can he get into the garbage?

    10. "No."

11. Has there been any recent trauma?

    11. "No."

12. Has your dog had any changes in mental attitude or personality?

    12. "He seems normal."

13. Do you have any other pets?

    13. "Nope."

14. Has your dog ever had a seizure?

    14. "Not that we've seen."

Go to Section B

Section B:

Which physical examination procedures would you perform at this time? *(Choose only the procedures you believe relevant to managing the case at this point.)*

15. Measure the body weight.

15. 15.2 kg. (He used to weigh 18 kg.)

16. Measure the rectal body temperature.

16. 37.9°C.

17. Take the pulse and heart rate.

17. The heart rate is 120 beats per minute; the pulse is strong and regular.

18. Measure the respiratory rate and note the character of respirations.

18. The respiratory rate is 24 per minute.

19. Auscultate the lungs.

19. Lung sounds are normal.

20. Auscultate the heart.

20. Heart sounds are normal.

21. Examine the oral cavity.

21. The oral cavity is normal; mucous membranes are pink; capillary refill time is 1 second.

22. Palpate the peripheral lymph nodes.

22. The lymph nodes are all firmer and larger than normal.

23. Palpate the abdomen.

23. Normal.

24. Examine the skin.

24. Normal.

25. Examine the ears, eyes, and nose.

25. No abnormalities.

26. Examine the neck and throat area.

26. Normal.

27. Assess cranial nerves, mental status, postural and spinal reflexes, gait and proprioception.

27. The dog is neurologically normal.

28. Palpate the muscles and bones, and flex and extend the joints.

28. The musculoskeletal system is normal.

Go to Section C

Section C:

Which diagnostic procedures would you perform? *(Choose only the procedures you believe relevant to managing the case at this point.)*

29. Collect blood for a complete blood count.

29. The complete blood count results show the following:
PCV = 42%
Hb = 13.2 g/dl
RBC = 7.5 million/mm^3
MCV = 68 fl

MCHC = 32 g/dl
MCH = 23 pg
WBC = 15,200/mm^3
Segs = 10,800/mm^3
Bands = 0/mm^3
Lymphocytes = 2200/mm^3
Monocytes = 200/mm^3
Eosinophils = 2000/mm^3
Basophils = 0/mm^3
Platelets = 295,000/mm^3
Total protein = 4.0 g/dl

30. Collect blood for a serum BUN and creatinine.

30. BUN = 18 mg/dl
Creatinine = 0.9 mg/dl

31. Collect blood for liver enzyme analysis.

31. ALT = 60 IU/L
GGT = 1 IU/L
SAP = 65 IU/L

32. Collect blood for serum total protein and albumin measurement.

32. Albumin = 1.8 g/dl
Total protein = 4.0 g/dl

33. Collect blood for serum calcium and phosphorus measurement.

33. Calcium = 8.6 mg/dl
Phosphorus = 4.6 mg/dl

34. Collect blood for serum amylase and lipase determination.

34. Amylase = 250 IU/L
Lipase = 100 IU/L

35. Collect blood for serum electrolyte quantitation.

35. Sodium = 145 mEq/L
Potassium = 4.4 mEq/L
Chloride = 112 mEq/L

36. Collect blood for serum blood glucose measurement.

36. Glucose = 105 mg/dl

37. Collect blood for serum cholesterol measurement.

37. Cholesterol = 100 mg/dl

38. Collect blood for serum bilirubin determination.

38. Total bilirubin = 0.1 mg/dl

39. Collect urine for a complete urinalysis.

39. The urine was collected by cystocentesis.
Color = yellow
Character = clear
Specific gravity = 1.035
pH = 6.5
Protein = negative
Glucose = negative
Ketones = negative
Bilirubin = 1+
Urobilinogen = negative
Blood = negative
WBC = 0-1/hpf
RBC = 3-5/hpf
Epithelial cells/hpf = occasionally
Bacteria = negative
Casts = negative
Crystals = negative

Sperm = negative
Fat = negative

40. Collect stool for fecal flotation.

40. Negative.

41. Obtain chest radiographs.

41. Normal.

42. Obtain abdominal radiographs.

42. Normal.

43. Perform a fine needle aspirate of the lymph nodes.

43. Eosinophilic lymphadenitis.

44. Collect stool for aerobic and anaerobic bacterial culture and antibiotic sensitivity.

44. Light growth of *E. coli,* sensitive to most antibiotics.

Go to Section D

Section D:

Considering the information you have gained so far, what further diagnostic tests would you like to perform? *(Choose only the tests you believe relevant to managing the case at this point.)*

45. Collect blood for fasting and postprandial serum bile acids determination.

45. Fasting serum bile acids = 5 mmol/L; postprandial serum bile acids = 6 mmol/L.

46. Administer barium and perform an upper gastrointestinal radiographic series.

46. Normal.

47. Examine a buffy coat smear.

47. No mast cells or microfilaria seen.

48. Collect blood for an occult heartworm test.

48. Negative.

49. Collect blood for immunoglobulin quantitation.

49. Normal.

50. Collect blood for trypsinlike immunoreactivity assay.

50. Results pending.

51. Collect blood for serum electrophoresis.

51. Normal.

52. Anesthetize the dog and collect bone marrow from the wing of the ilium.

52. Normal.

53. Ultrasound the abdomen.

53. Normal.

54. Anesthetize the dog and perform an upper gastrointestinal endoscopy.

54. The stomach is grossly normal; duodenum is red and bleeds easily. Biopsies are consistent with severe eosinophilic enteritis.

55. Collect blood pre- and post-ACTH administration for serum cortisol determination.

55. Pre-ACTH cortisol = 3.4 µg/dl; post-ACTH cortisol = 14.1 µg/dl.

56. Perform a rectal scraping and examine for the presence of *Histoplasma capsulatum.*

56. No abnormalities.

Section E:

Which course of action would you take? *(Choose only one.)*

57. Prescribe prednisone at physiological doses.	57. End of problem.
58. Prescribe pancreatic enzyme replacement and recheck the dog in 2 weeks.	58. End of problem.
59. Treat the dog with fenbendazole, followed by metronidazole, and prescribe a hypoallergenic diet. Reexamine the dog in 3 weeks.	59. End of problem.
60. Recommend euthanasia due to the poor prognosis.	60. End of problem.
61. Prescribe cephalexin and schedule a recheck examination in 2 weeks.	61. End of problem.
62. Prescribe a high quality, high protein diet and advise the owner to weigh the dog at weekly intervals.	62. End of problem.

END OF PROBLEM

Opening Scene:

The owner of a 7-year-old neutered male domestic shorthair cat presents her cat to you with an ocular discharge for 2 days. Two nights ago, he was out all night, and when he came home he was squinting his left eye. The discharge from the eye is clear and watery. The right eye seems fine. He is an indoor and outdoor cat who lives in the midwestern United States and has not traveled. He is current on his vaccinations, including rabies.

Go to Section A

Section A:

What questions would you like to ask the owner? *(Choose only the questions you believe relevant to managing the case at this point.)*

1. Does he fight with other cats?	1. "He has been known to fight but not recently that I know of."
2. Has he had ocular disease before?	2. "No."
3. Does he have any wounds?	3. "Not that I've seen."
4. Is there a possibility of toxin exposure?	4. "Well, he goes outside and I don't really know what he could get into."
5. Has he had any previous illnesses, injuries, or surgeries?	5. "No, only his neuter surgery at a year of age."
6. What is his diet and how much does he eat daily?	6. "He eats dry commercial cat food, about one half to three fourths of a cup a day. His appetite is fine."
7. Has your cat been sneezing or coughing?	7. "No."
8. Has your cat been vomiting or had any diarrhea?	8. "No."
9. Do you have other animals, and if so, are they sick?	9. "Yes, we have one other cat, too, but she seems fine."
10. Has there been any change in his thirst or urination habits?	10. "No."
11. Has your cat collapsed or had any seizures?	11. "Not that I have seen."
12. Has your cat had any changes in mental attitude or personality?	12. "His attitude is a little off; maybe he's a bit quiet for him."
13. Does your cat have any skin disease?	13. "No."

Section B:

Which physical examination procedures would you perform at this time? *(Choose only the procedures you believe relevant to managing the case at this point.)*

14. Measure the body weight.	14. 4.5 kg.
15. Measure the rectal body temperature.	15. 38.3°C.
16. Take the pulse and heart rate.	16. The heart rate is 144 beats per minute; the pulse is strong and regular.
17. Measure the respiratory rate and note the character of respirations.	17. The respiratory rate is 16 per minute.
18. Auscultate the lungs.	18. Lung sounds are normal.
19. Auscultate the heart.	19. Heart sounds are normal.
20. Examine the oral cavity.	20. Mucous membranes are pink, capillary refill time is 1 second; no oral lesions.
21. Palpate the peripheral lymph nodes.	21. Normal.
22. Palpate the abdomen.	22. Normal.
23. Examine the skin.	23. Normal.
24. Examine the ears and nose.	24. No abnormalities.
25. Examine the external features of the right eye.	25. Normal.
26. Examine the external features of the left eye.	26. The left pupil is smaller than the right; the anterior chamber is hazy (aqueous flare); the cornea is cloudy and the conjunctival and episcleral blood vessels are hyperemic.
27. Assess cranial nerves, mental status, postural and spinal reflexes, gait and proprioception.	27. The nervous system is normal.
28. Palpate the muscles and bones, and flex and extend the joints.	28. No abnormalities.

Go to Section C

Section C:

Which diagnostic procedures would you perform? *(Choose only the procedures you believe relevant to managing the case at this point.)*

29. Collect blood for a complete blood count.

29. The complete blood count results show the following:
PCV = 42%
Hb = 18.2 g/dl
RBC = 11.5 million/mm^3
MCV = 42 fl
MCHC = 33 g/dl
MCH = 15 pg
WBC = 12,800/mm^3
Segs = 10,800/mm^3
Bands = 0/mm^3
Lymphocytes = 1800/mm^3
Monocytes = 100/mm^3
Eosinophils = 100/mm^3
Basophils = 0/mm^3
Platelets = 310,000/mm^3
Total protein = 7.2 g/dl

30. Collect blood for a serum glucose concentration.

30. Glucose = 105 mg/dl

31. Collect blood for a BUN and creatinine determination.

31. BUN = 16 mg/dl
Creatinine = 1.0 mg/dl

32. Collect blood for serum liver enzyme measurement.

32. ALT = 60 IU/L
GGT = 1 IU/L
SAP = 65 IU/L

33. Collect blood for calcium and phosphorus determination.

33. Calcium = 9.6 mg/dl
Phosphorus = 3.6 mg/dl

34. Collect blood for serum cholesterol measurement.

34. Cholesterol = 124 mg/dl

35. Collect urine for a urinalysis.

35. The urine was collected free catch.
Color = yellow
Character = clear
Specific gravity = 1.048
pH = 6.5
Protein = negative
Glucose = negative
Ketones = negative
Bilirubin = negative
Urobilinogen = negative
Blood = 2+
WBC = 1-3/hpf
RBC = 5-10/hpf
Epithelial cells/hpf = occasionally

Bacteria = negative
Casts = negative
Crystals = negative
Sperm = negative
Fat = negative

36. Collect blood for a serum thyroid hormone concentration.

37. Obtain a conjunctival scraping.

38. Collect blood for a feline leukemia virus test.

39. Collect blood for a feline immunodeficiency virus test.

40. Perform a Schirmer tear test on both eyes.

41. Stain the cornea of the left eye with fluorescein.

42. Perform a funduscopic examination on the right and left eyes.

43. Sedate the cat and flush the tear duct of the left eye.

44. Instill topical anesthetic in the left eye and inspect behind the third eyelid.

45. Instill topical anesthetic in the left eye and measure the intraocular pressure.

36. Serum thyroxine = 2.0 µg/dl

37. Suppurative inflammation; no etiologic agent identified.

38. Negative.

39. Negative.

40. Tear production—OD = 20 mm/minute; OS = 24 mm/minute.

41. Negative.

42. The right eye is normal; the cloudiness of the left anterior chamber precludes assessment of the left fundus.

43. The tear duct is patent.

44. No lesions or foreign bodies identified behind the third eyelid.

45. Intraocular pressure—OD = 20 mm Hg; OS = 12 mm Hg.

Go to Section D

Section D:

Considering the information you have gained so far, what further diagnostic tests would you like to perform? (*Choose only the tests you believe relevant to managing the case at this point.*)

46. Collect blood for *Cryptococcus neoformans* serology.

47. Collect blood for herpes serology.

48. Anesthetize the cat and perform aqueocentesis for cytology and a *Toxoplasma* titer.

49. Obtain chest radiographs.

50. Obtain abdominal radiographs.

51. Instill 10% phenylephrine in the eyes and note the change in pupil size.

46. <1:2.

47. <1:2.

48. Suppurative inflammation; no organisms seen. *Toxoplasma* specific antibody production is present within the aqueous.

49. Normal.

50. Normal.

51. No dilation of both pupils.

52. Instill 1% hydroxyamphetamine in the eyes and note the change in pupil size.

52. Dilation of both pupils.

53. Collect blood for *Toxoplasma* serology.

53. IgG = 1:512; IgM = 1:1024.

54. Collect blood for feline infectious peritonitis virus serology.

54. 1:100.

55. Anesthetize the cat for skull radiographs.

55. No abnormal findings.

Go to Section E

Section E:

Which course of action would you take? *(Choose only one.)*

56. Administer mannitol intravenously at an appropriate dose and prescribe pilocarpine ophthalmic drops. Schedule a recheck examination in 2 days.

56. End of problem.

57. Prescribe prednisone and atropine ophthalmic solutions and oral clindamycin therapy and schedule a recheck examination in 1 week.

57. End of problem.

58. Recommend euthanasia due to the risk of transmission of this disease to the owner.

58. End of problem.

59. Anesthetize the cat and perform an enucleation of the left eye.

59. End of problem.

60. Anesthetize the cat and perform a third eyelid flap. Prescribe a topical antibiotic ointment and schedule a recheck examination in 1 week.

60. End of problem.

61. Prescribe tetracycline ophthalmic ointment for 2 weeks.

61. End of problem.

END OF PROBLEM

Opening Scene:

The owner of a 2-year-old female Labrador retriever presents the dog to you with complaints that it has exhibited exercise intolerance over the past few weeks. The dog usually is very active and plays constantly with the kids. Yesterday, while chasing them on their bikes, she just collapsed. After a rest, she was fine again. She lives in the western United States and has not traveled. She is up to date on her vaccinations, including distemper/parvovirus and rabies and is on monthly heartworm preventative.

Go to Section A

Section A:

What questions would you like to ask the owner? (*Choose only the questions you believe relevant to managing the case at this point.*)

1. Has she had any previous illnesses, injuries, or surgeries?

    1. "She has been a healthy dog until now."

2. Has there been any change in her thirst or urinary habits?

    2. "She does seem to drink more and urinate larger volumes over the past few months."

3. Is she currently taking any medications?

    3. "No."

4. What diet does she normally eat and about how much does she consume in a day?

    4. "She eats a premium dry dog food. She usually eats about 4 cups daily."

5. Describe the episode of collapse.

    5. "It's the only time she's ever done it, and I was scared she was dying. She was running with the kids and suddenly stumbled and fell to her side. She laid there quietly for a minute or so and then eventually got up and acted fine. She was real limp when she collapsed."

6. Is your dog lame?

    6. "Not that I've noticed."

7. Does she vomit or have diarrhea?

    7. "No."

8. Has she been coughing or sneezing?

    8. "No."

9. Has she had any difficulty breathing?

    9. "She seems to breathe hard when she exercises, but otherwise she's fine."

10. Is there any possibility of toxin exposure?

    10. "No."

11. Has there been any recent trauma?

    11. "No."

12. Has your dog had any changes in mental attitude or personality?

    12. "No."

13. When was her last heat? Has she ever had puppies?

    13. Her last heat was 3 months ago. She has never been bred."

14. Has your dog ever had a seizure?

    14. "Not that we've seen."

Go to Section B

Section B:

Which physical examination procedures would you perform at this time? (*Choose only the procedures you believe relevant to managing the case at this point.*)

15. Measure the body weight.

15. 32.2 kg.

16. Measure the rectal body temperature.

16. 37.9°C.

17. Take the pulse and heart rate.

17. The heart rate is 168 beats per minute; the pulse is strong and regular.

18. Measure the respiratory rate and note the character of respirations.

18. The respiratory rate is 60 per minute.

19. Auscultate the lungs.

19. Lung sounds are normal.

20. Auscultate the heart.

20. There is a grade II systolic ejection murmur with a point of maximal intensity at the left base.

21. Examine the oral cavity.

21. The oral cavity is normal; mucous membranes are dark red; capillary refill time is 1 second.

22. Palpate the peripheral lymph nodes.

22. Normal.

23. Palpate the abdomen.

23. Normal.

24. Examine the skin.

24. Normal.

25. Examine the ears, eyes, and nose.

25. No abnormalities.

26. Examine the neck and throat area.

26. Normal.

27. Assess cranial nerves, mental status, postural and spinal reflexes, gait and proprioception.

27. The dog is neurologically normal.

28. Palpate the muscles and bones, and flex and extend the joints.

28. The musculoskeletal system is normal.

Go to Section C

Section C:

Which diagnostic procedures would you perform? (*Choose only the procedures you believe relevant to managing the case at this point.*)

29. Collect blood for a complete blood count.

29. The complete blood count results show the following:
PCV = 78%
Hb = 23.2 g/dl
RBC = 14.5 million/mm^3
MCV = 58 fl
MCHC = 32 g/dl

MCH = 23 pg
WBC = 9800/mm^3
Segs = 6800/mm^3
Bands = 0/mm^3
Lymphocytes = 2200/mm^3
Monocytes = 200/mm^3
Eosinophils = 600/mm^3
Basophils = 0/mm^3
Platelets = 245,000/mm^3
Total protein = 6.5 g/dl

30. Collect blood for a serum BUN and creatinine determination.

30. BUN = 18 mg/dl
Creatinine = 1.6 mg/dl

31. Collect blood for liver enzyme analysis.

31. ALT = 60 IU/L
GGT = 1 IU/L
SAP = 65 IU/L

32. Collect blood for serum total protein and albumin measurement.

32. Albumin = 3.5 g/dl
Total protein = 6.5 g/dl

33. Collect blood for serum calcium and phosphorus measurement.

33. Calcium = 10.6 mg/dl
Phosphorus = 3.6 mg/dl

34. Collect blood for serum amylase and lipase determination.

34. Amylase = 250 IU/L
Lipase = 100 IU/L

35. Collect blood for serum electrolyte quantitation.

35. Sodium = 145 mEq/L
Potassium = 4.4 mEq/L
Chloride = 112 mEq/L

36. Collect blood for serum blood glucose measurement.

36. Glucose = 105 mg/dl.

37. Collect blood for serum cholesterol measurement.

37 Cholesterol = 100 mg/dl.

38. Collect blood for serum bilirubin determination.

38. Total bilirubin = 0.1 mg/dl.

39. Collect urine for a complete urinalysis.

39. The urine was collected by cystocentesis.
Color = yellow
Character = clear
Specific gravity = 1.012
pH = 7.5
Protein = negative
Glucose = negative
Ketones = negative
Bilirubin = negative
Urobilinogen = negative
Blood = negative
WBC = 0-1/hpf
RBC = 3-5/hpf
Epithelial cells/hpf = occasionally
Bacteria = negative
Casts = negative
Crystals = negative

40. Collect an arterial blood gas sample for analysis.

40. The results of the arterial blood gas analysis show the following:
    pH = 7.24
    pO_2 = 76 mm Hg
    pCO_2 = 25 mm Hg
    HCO_3 = 12 mEq/L

41. Obtain chest radiographs.

41. Lungs are normal; pulmonary vasculature appears mildly undercirculated; cardiomegaly is apparent.

42. Obtain abdominal radiographs.

42. Normal.

43. Exercise the dog and observe for collapse.

43. The dog collapses after 5 minutes of strenuous exercise; it is most consistent with a syncopal episode.

44. Perform an electrocardiogram.

44. Sinus tachycardia with evidence of right ventricular hypertrophy.

Go to Section D

Section D:

Considering the information you have gained so far, what further diagnostic tests would you like to perform? *(Choose only the tests you believe relevant to managing the case at this point.)*

45. Collect blood for plasma erythropoietin measurement.

45. Pending.

46. Anesthetize the dog and collect muscle biopsies.

46. Normal.

47. Anesthetize the dog for cerebrospinal fluid collection.

47. Normal.

48. Perform a Tensilon response test.

48. There is no difference in the dog's response to Tensilon versus no treatment after collapse.

49. Perform an echocardiogram.

49. Malposition of the aortic root, right ventricular hypertrophy, and a ventricular septal defect are identified and consistent with a tetralogy of Fallot.

50. Collect blood for antiacetylcholine receptor antibody testing.

50. Results pending.

51. Ultrasound the abdomen.

51. No abnormalities noted.

52. Anesthetize the dog for an ultrasound-guided renal biopsy.

52. Normal renal tissue.

53. Anesthetize the dog for selective angiography.

53. Findings are consistent with a tetralogy of Fallot.

54. Perform an electrocardiogram and collect blood after exercise for blood gas, glucose, and potassium analysis.

54. All values are within normal limits with the exception of mild metabolic acidosis.

55. Collect blood pre- and post-ACTH administration for serum cortisol determination.

55. Pre-ACTH cortisol = 3.2 µg/dl; post-ACTH cortisol = 14.4 µg/dl.

56. Collect blood for thyroid hormone analysis.

56. T_4 = 3.2 µg/dl.

57. Sedate the dog and collect bone marrow from the iliac crest.

57. Normal bone marrow with erythroid hyperplasia.

Go to Section E

Section E:

Which course of action would you take? *(Choose only one.)*

58. Prescribe hydroxyurea and schedule a recheck examination in 2 weeks.

58. End of problem.

59. Perform a phlebotomy, remove 500 ml of blood, and prescribe beta blocker therapy.

59. End of problem.

60. Prescribe pyridostigmine and schedule a recheck examination in 2 weeks.

60. End of problem.

61. Recommend an exploratory laparotomy for removal of a kidney.

61. End of problem.

62. Refer the dog to a specialist for further workup.

62. End of problem.

63. Administer intravenous fluids to replace the deficit and supply maintenance requirements.

63. End of problem.

END OF PROBLEM

PROBLEM 41

Opening Scene:

The owner of a 1-year-old neutered male domestic shorthaired cat presents the cat to you at your exclusive small animal practice with a problem of vomiting and anorexia for 2 days. The cat usually eats dry cat food. The owner has offered him canned cat foods, but he refuses everything, even fresh tuna. He is an indoor cat and current on his vaccinations, including rabies.

Go to Section A

Section A:

What questions would you like to ask the owner? (*Choose only the questions you believe relevant to managing the case at this point.*)

1. What does the vomitus look like?

1. "It began as food, semi-digested, but now is just a yellow foam."

2. Approximately how many times has he vomited?

2. "He has vomited eight to 10 times in the last 2 days."

3. Has your cat had any diarrhea?

3. "No, he hasn't passed any stool in 2 days. Before that it was normal."

4. Is there a possibility of exposure to toxins, such as house plants or insecticides?

4. "We have a variety of house plants, but I have never seen him eat any of them. We did spray him for fleas 10 days ago."

5. Has he had any previous illnesses, injuries, or surgeries?

5. "No, only his neuter surgery at 6 months of age."

6. Is he currently taking any medications?

6. "No."

7. Do you have other animals and, if so, are they ill?

7. "We have another cat that is 3 years old. She is not sick, though."

8. Has he been sneezing or coughing or had any nasal discharge?

8. "No."

9. Has your cat lost weight?

9. "Not that I can appreciate."

10. Has there been any change in his thirst or urination habits?

10. "He is not drinking much at all and has only urinated once since yesterday."

11. Does your cat ever play with thread or string?

11. "Well, I am a quilter so I guess he could get threads, but I do try to be careful."

12. Has your cat had any changes in mental attitude or personality?

12. "He's very quiet and has started hiding."

13. Does your cat have any skin disease?

13. "No."

Go to Section B

Section B:

Which physical examination procedures would you perform at this time? *(Choose only the procedures you believe relevant to managing the case at this point.)*

14. Measure the body weight.

14. 5.2 kg.

15. Measure the rectal body temperature.

15. 40.3°C.

16. Take the pulse and heart rate.

16. The heart rate is 180 beats per minute; the pulse is strong and regular.

17. Measure the respiratory rate and note the character of respirations.

17. The respiratory rate is 16 per minute.

18. Auscultate the lungs.

18. Lung sounds are normal.

19. Auscultate the heart.

19. Heart sounds are normal.

20. Examine the oral cavity.

20. Mucous membranes are pale pink; capillary refill time is 2 seconds.

21. Palpate the peripheral lymph nodes.

21. Normal.

22. Palpate the abdomen.

22. The cat resents palpation; however, no obvious abnormalities are noted.

23. Examine the skin.

23. Normal.

24. Examine the ears, eyes, and nose.

24. No abnormalities.

25. Assess the hydration status.

25. The skin turgor is decreased and the mucous membranes are dry; the cat is estimated to be 7% dehydrated.

26. Assess cranial nerves, mental status, postural and spinal reflexes, gait and proprioception.

26. The cat is neurologically normal.

27. Palpate the muscles and bones, and flex and extend the joints.

27. The musculoskeletal system is normal.

28. Examine the area under the tongue.

28. A string is noted under the tongue.

Go to Section C

Section C:

Which diagnostic procedures would you perform? *(Choose only the procedures you believe relevant to managing the case at this point.)*

29. Collect blood for a complete blood count.

29. The complete blood count results show the following:
PCV = 42%
Hb = 18.2 g/dl

RBC = 11.5 million/mm^3
MCV = 42 fl
MCHC = 33 g/dl
MCH = 15 pg
WBC = 23,800/mm^3
Segs = 21,600/mm^3
Bands = 1200/mm^3
Lymphocytes = 400/mm^3
Monocytes = 600/mm^3
Eosinophils = 0/mm^3
Basophils = 0/mm^3
Platelets = 320,000/mm^3
Total protein = 6.2 g/dl

30. Collect blood for a serum glucose concentration.

30. Glucose = 185 mg/dl

31. Collect blood for a BUN and creatinine determination.

31. BUN = 66 mg/dl
Creatinine = 3.0 mg/dl

32. Collect blood for serum liver enzyme measurement.

32. ALT = 60 IU/L
GGT = 2 IU/L
SAP = 65 IU/L

33. Collect blood for calcium and phosphorus determination.

33. Calcium = 9.6 mg/dl
Phosphorus = 3.6 mg/dl

34. Collect blood for serum electrolytes measurement.

34. Sodium = 134 mEq/L
Potassium = 3.2 mEq/L
Chloride = 106 mEq/L

35. Collect blood for serum bilirubin measurement.

35. Bilirubin = 0.6 mg/dl.

36. Collect blood for a serum thyroid hormone concentration.

36. Serum thyroxine = 2.0 μg/dl.

37. Collect urine for a urinalysis.

37. The urine was collected free catch.
Color = dark yellow
Character = clear
Specific gravity = 1.068
pH = 6.5
Protein = negative
Glucose = negative
Ketones = negative
Bilirubin = negative
Urobilinogen = negative
Blood = negative
WBC/hpf = rare
RBC/hpf = rare
Epithelial cells/hpf = occasionally
Bacteria = negative
Casts = negative
Crystals = negative
Sperm = negative
Fat = negative

38. Collect blood for a feline leukemia virus test.

38. Negative.

39. Collect blood for a feline immunodeficiency virus test.

40. Collect stool for fecal flotation.

41. Obtain chest radiographs.

42. Obtain abdominal radiographs.

43. Perform an abdominocentesis to collect peritoneal fluid for cytology.

44. Perform an upper gastrointestinal study with barium.

45. Collect blood for serum amylase and lipase determination.

39. Negative.

40. Negative.

41. Normal.

42. The abdominal detail is poor; however, it is apparent that the intestines are plicated.

43. About 1 ml of a sanguinous fluid is removed easily from the abdomen. Cytologically, there are 90% degenerative neutrophils and 10% mononuclear cells. No bacteria are noted.

44. The cat vomits the contrast media, and the study cannot be completed.

45. Amylase = 200 IU/L
Lipase = 100 IU/L

Go to Section D

Section D:

Considering the information you have gained so far, what further diagnostic tests/therapeutic measures would you like to perform? (*Choose only the tests you believe relevant to managing the case at this point.*)

46. Collect blood for feline infectious peritonitis serology.

47. Collect fasting and postprandial blood samples for serum bile acid analysis.

48. Perform a 24-hour creatinine clearance.

49. Perform a funduscopic examination.

50. Collect blood before and after administration of ACTH for serum cortisol analysis.

51. Ultrasound the abdomen.

52. Place an intravenous catheter and administer deficit and maintenance fluids.

53. Collect blood for *Toxoplasma* serology.

54. Place an intravenous catheter and administer broad spectrum antibiotics.

55. Anesthetize the cat for endoscopic examination and gastrointestinal biopsies.

56. Anesthetize the cat for renal biopsy.

46. 1:100.

47. Fasting serum bile acids = 5 mmol/L; postprandial serum bile acids = 8 mmol/L.

48. 2.8 ml/minute/kg.

49. Normal.

50. Pre-ACTH cortisol = 2.8 μg/dl; post-ACTH cortisol = 14.2 μg/dl.

51. Normal.

52. Done. The cat's overall status improves.

53. IgG = 1:4; IgM = 1:4.

54. Done.

55. The stomach and duodenum are diffusely reddened. Biopsies pending.

56. Normal.

Section E:

Which course of action would you take? *(Choose only one.)*

57. Prescribe a broad spectrum anthelmintic and a hypoallergenic diet; schedule a recheck examination in 1 week.

    57. End of problem.

58. Refer the cat to a specialist for further workup.

    58. End of problem.

59. Prescribe amoxicillin and schedule a recheck examination in 2 weeks.

    59. End of problem.

60. Prescribe prednisone, metronidazole, and a hypoallergenic diet and reexamine the cat in 1 week.

    60. End of problem.

61. Recommend that the owners withhold food for 24 hours, then begin a bland diet of hamburger and rice.

    61. End of problem.

62. Bathe the cat and tell the owners that he will be fine now that the insecticide is washed off.

    62. End of problem.

63. Schedule the cat for an exploratory laparotomy as soon as he is stabilized.

    63. End of problem.

END OF PROBLEM

PROBLEM 42

Opening Scene:

The owner of a 3-year-old spayed female Cocker spaniel presents the dog to you at your mixed animal practice with a complaint that the dog has been lethargic for the past 2 days. Also, the dog is not eating anything the owner offers her. She lives in the midwestern United States and has not traveled. She is up to date on her vaccinations, including distemper/parvovirus and rabies and is on monthly heartworm preventative.

Go to Section A

Section A:

What questions would you like to ask the owner? (*Choose only the questions you believe relevant to managing the case at this point.*)

1. Has she had any previous illnesses, injuries, or surgeries?

2. Has there been any change in her thirst or urinary habits?

3. Is she currently on any medications?

4. What diet does she normally eat and about how much does she consume in a day?

5. Is your dog weak or has she ever collapsed?

6. Is she an indoor or outdoor dog?

7. Has she vomited or had any diarrhea?

8. Has she been coughing, sneezing, or had any nasal discharge?

9. Has she had any difficulty breathing?

10. Is there any possibility of toxin exposure?

11. Is your dog lame?

12. When was she last vaccinated?

13. Do you have any other pets and, if so, are they ill?

14. Has your dog had a seizure or a change in personality?

1. "She was spayed at 6 months of age; otherwise she's been fine."

2. "No changes."

3. "No."

4. "She eats a premium dry dog food, free choice, about 1½ cups a day."

5. "She seems weak today, but she hasn't collapsed."

6. "She's an indoor dog. She only goes out in our fenced-in yard."

7. "No."

8. "No."

9. "No."

10. "No."

11. "No."

12. "About 1 month ago."

13. "Yes, we have a cat but she's fine."

14. "Not that we've noticed."

Go to Section B

Section B:

Which physical examination procedures would you perform at this time? *(Choose only the procedures you believe relevant to managing the case at this point.)*

15. Measure the body weight.

15. 12.2 kg.

16. Measure the rectal body temperature.

16. 40.2°C.

17. Take the pulse and heart rate.

17. The heart rate is 180 beats per minute; the pulse is strong and regular.

18. Measure the respiratory rate and note the character of respirations.

18. The respiratory rate is 48 per minute.

19. Auscultate the lungs.

19. Lung sounds are normal.

20. Auscultate the heart.

20. There is a grade I holosystolic heart murmur over the left base.

21. Examine the oral cavity.

21. The oral cavity is normal; mucous membranes are pale pink and icteric; capillary refill time is 1 second.

22. Palpate the peripheral lymph nodes.

22. Normal.

23. Palpate the abdomen.

23. The spleen and liver are mildly enlarged.

24. Examine the skin.

24. Normal.

25. Examine the ears, eyes, and nose.

25. No abnormalities except icterus is noted in the sclera.

26. Examine the neck and throat area.

26. Normal.

27. Assess cranial nerves, mental status, postural and spinal reflexes, gait and proprioception.

27. The dog is neurologically normal.

28. Palpate the muscles and bones, and flex and extend the joints.

28. The musculoskeletal system is normal.

29. Evaluate the hydration status.

29. The dog appears about 5% dehydrated.

Go to Section C

Section C:

Which diagnostic procedures would you perform? *(Choose only the procedures you believe relevant to managing the case at this point.)*

30. Collect blood for a complete blood count.

30. The complete blood count results show the following:
PCV = 18%
Hb = 6.2 g/dl

RBC = 4.5 million/mm^3
MCV = 78 fl
MCHC = 32 g/dl
MCH = 23 pg
WBC = 30,000/mm^3
Segs = 27,000/mm^3
Bands = 800/mm^3
Lymphocytes = 1200/mm^3
Monocytes = 400/mm^3
Eosinophils = 600/mm3
Basophils = 0/mm^3
Platelets = 185,000/mm^3
Total protein = 7.0 g/dl
Comments: 3+ spherocytosis, 3+ polychro-
masia, 4+ anisocytosis.

31. Collect blood for a serum BUN and creatinine determination.

31. BUN = 58 mg/dl
Creatinine = 2.6 mg/dl

32. Collect blood for liver enzyme analysis.

32. ALT = 260 IU/L
GGT = 1 IU/L
SAP = 265 IU/L

33. Collect blood for serum total protein and albumin measurement.

33. Albumin = 4.3 g/dl
Total protein = 7.0 g/dl

34. Collect blood for serum calcium and phosphorus measurement.

34. Calcium = 10.6 mg/dl
Phosphorus = 4.6 mg/dl

35. Collect blood for serum amylase and lipase determination.

35. Amylase = 250 IU/L
Lipase = 100 IU/L

36. Collect blood for serum electrolyte quantitation.

36. Sodium = 145 mEq/L
Potassium = 4.4 mEq/L
Chloride = 108 mEq/L

37. Collect blood for serum blood glucose measurement.

37. Glucose = 105 mg/dl.

38. Collect blood for serum cholesterol measurement.

38. Cholesterol = 100 mg/dl.

39. Collect blood for serum bilirubin determination.

39. Total bilirubin = 4.1 mg/dl.

40. Collect urine for a complete urinalysis.

40. The urine was collected by cystocentesis.
Color = dark yellow
Character = clear
Specific gravity = 1.047
pH = 6.5
Protein = negative
Glucose = negative
Ketones = negative
Bilirubin = 3+
Urobilinogen = negative
Blood = negative
WBC = 0-1/hpf
RBC = 3-5/hpf

Epithelial cells/hpf = occasionally
Bacteria = negative
Casts = negative
Crystals = negative
Sperm = negative
Fat = negative

41. Collect stool for fecal flotation.

41. Negative.

42. Obtain chest radiographs.

42. Normal.

43. Obtain abdominal radiographs.

43. Mild hepatosplenomegaly; no other abnormalities noted.

44. Collect blood for a reticulocyte count.

44. Reticulocytes = 12%.

45. Perform an electrocardiogram.

45. Sinus tachycardia.

Go to Section D

Section D:

Considering the information you have gained so far, what further diagnostic tests/therapeutic measures would you like to perform? *(Choose only the tests you believe relevant to managing the case at this point.)*

46. Collect blood for fasting and postprandial serum bile acids determination.

46. Fasting serum bile acids = 45 mmol/L; postprandial serum bile acids = 56 mmol/L.

47. Sedate the dog for collection of bone marrow from the iliac crest.

47. Erythroid and myeloid hyperplasia; erythrophagocytosis noted.

48. Administer barium sulfate and perform an upper gastrointestinal radiographic series.

48. Normal.

49. Administer a whole blood transfusion.

49. Done.

50. Perform an echocardiogram.

50. No abnormal findings.

51. Collect blood for a Coomb's test.

51. Positive.

52. Collect blood for an antinuclear antibody test.

52. Negative.

53. Sedate the dog and perform arthrocentesis.

53. Normal joint fluid.

54. Collect blood and perform a direct slide agglutination test.

54. No erythrocyte agglutination is noted in saline.

55. Ultrasound the abdomen.

55. No abnormal findings other than mild hepatosplenomegaly.

56. Perform abdominocentesis for the purpose of obtaining a sample of abdominal fluid.

56. No fluid obtained.

57. Perform an ultrasound-guided liver biopsy.

57. Results pending.

58. Collect blood for assessment of coagulation parameters.

58. Activated clotting time = 100 seconds (normal = 90-120 seconds); activated partial thromboplastin time = 14 seconds (normal = 12-18 seconds); prothrombin time = 8 seconds (normal = 6-10 seconds); platelets = 190,000/mm^3.

Go to Section E

Section E:

Which course of action would you take? (*Choose only one.*)

59. Prescribe broad spectrum antibiotics and schedule a recheck examination in 2 days.

59. End of problem.

60. Prescribe an immunosuppressive dose of prednisone, administer fluids, and reevaluate the PCV daily.

60. End of problem.

61. Prescribe vitamin K therapy and reevaluate the PCV in 2 days.

61. End of problem.

62. Prescribe a homemade diet and schedule a recheck examination in 1 week.

62. End of problem.

63. Refer the dog to a specialist for further workup.

63. End of problem.

64. Prescribe a protein-restricted diet and give the owners a poor prognosis.

64. End of problem.

END OF PROBLEM

Opening Scene:

The owner of a 5-year-old spayed female golden retriever presents the dog to you at your mixed animal practice with a complaint that the dog has been lethargic for the past 2 months. Also, the dog has gained weight recently. Her normal weight has been 32 kg in the past. She lives in the midwestern United States and has not traveled. She is up to date on her vaccinations, including distemper/parvovirus and rabies and is on monthly heartworm preventative.

Go to Section A

Section A:

What questions would you like to ask the owner? (*Choose only the questions you believe relevant to managing the case at this point.*)

1. Has she had any previous illnesses, injuries, or surgeries?

    1. "She was spayed at 6 months of age; otherwise she's been fine."

2. Has there been any change in her thirst or urinary habits?

    2. "No changes."

3. Is she currently on any medications?

    3. "No."

4. What diet does she normally eat and about how much does she consume in a day?

    4. "She eats a premium dry dog food, free choice, about 1½ cups a day."

5. Do you give her treats between meals?

    5. "She gets two small dog bones daily."

6. Have you noticed any problems with her skin?

    6. "Her coat is thin over her back and her tail is practically hairless."

7. Has she vomited or had any diarrhea?

    7. "No."

8. Has she been coughing, sneezing, or had any nasal discharge?

    8. "No."

9. Has she had any difficulty breathing?

    9. "No."

10. Has there been a recent change in her feeding or exercise routine?

    10. "No."

11. Does your dog scratch herself excessively?

    11. "No."

12. Is your dog weak or has she ever collapsed?

    12. "She's not really weak, but she does lay around more than usual."

13. Do you have any other pets and, if so, are they ill?

    13. "Yes, we have a cat but she's fine."

14. Has your dog had a seizure or a change in personality?

    14. "Not that we've noticed."

Section B:

Which physical examination procedures would you perform at this time? *(Choose only the procedures you believe relevant to managing the case at this point.)*

15. Measure the body weight.	15. 36.8 kg.
16. Measure the rectal body temperature.	16. 38.2°C.
17. Take the pulse and heart rate.	17. The heart rate is 60 beats per minute; the pulse is strong and regular.
18. Measure the respiratory rate and note the character of respirations.	18. The respiratory rate is 18 per minute.
19. Auscultate the lungs.	19. Lung sounds are normal.
20. Auscultate the heart.	20. Heart sounds are normal.
21. Examine the oral cavity.	21. The oral cavity is normal; mucous membranes are pink; capillary refill time is 1 second.
22. Palpate the peripheral lymph nodes.	22. Normal.
23. Palpate the abdomen.	23. Normal.
24. Examine the skin.	24. There is a bilaterally symmetrical loss of guard hairs over the trunk and flanks. The tail has very sparse hair growth. The skin is generally hyperpigmented, especially in the inguinal region.
25. Examine the ears, eyes, and nose.	25. No abnormalities.
26. Examine the neck and throat area.	26. Normal except for a bilateral ceruminous otitis externa.
27. Assess cranial nerves, mental status, postural and spinal reflexes, gait and proprioception.	27. The dog is neurologically normal.
28. Palpate the muscles and bones, and flex and extend the joints.	28. The musculoskeletal system is normal.
29. Evaluate the hydration status.	29. The dog appears normally hydrated.

Section C:

Which diagnostic procedures would you perform? *(Choose only the procedures you believe relevant to managing the case at this point.)*

30. Collect blood for a complete blood count.

30. The complete blood count results show the following:
PCV = 28%
Hb = 10.2 g/dl
RBC = 4.5 million/mm^3
MCV = 70 fl
MCHC = 32 g/dl
MCH = 23 pg
WBC = 10,000/mm^3
Segs = 8000/mm^3
Bands = 0/mm^3
Lymphocytes = 1000/mm^3
Monocytes = 400/mm^3
Eosinophils = 600/mm^3
Basophils = 0/mm^3
Platelets = 285,000/mm^3
Total protein = 7.0 g/dl

31. Collect blood for a serum BUN and creatinine determination.

31. BUN = 18 mg/dl
Creatinine = 1.2 mg/dl

32. Collect blood for liver enzyme analysis.

32. ALT = 120 IU/L
GGT = 4 IU/L
SAP = 265 IU/L

33. Collect blood for serum total protein and albumin measurement.

33. Albumin = 4.3 g/dl
Total protein = 7.0 g/dl

34. Collect blood for serum calcium and phosphorus measurement.

34. Calcium = 10.6 mg/dl
Phosphorus = 4.6 mg/dl

35. Collect blood for serum amylase and lipase determination.

35. Amylase = 250 IU/L
Lipase = 100 IU/L

36. Collect blood for serum electrolyte quantitation.

36. Sodium = 145 mEq/L
Potassium = 4.4 mEq/L
Chloride = 108 mEq/L

37. Collect blood for serum blood glucose measurement.

37. Glucose = 105 mg/dl

38. Collect blood for serum cholesterol measurement.

38. Cholesterol = 650 mg/dl

39. Collect blood for serum bilirubin determination.

39. Total bilirubin = 0.1 mg/dl

40. Collect urine for a complete urinalysis.

40. The urine was collected by cystocentesis.
Color = dark yellow
Character = clear
Specific gravity = 1.047

pH = 6.5
Protein = negative
Glucose = negative
Ketones = negative
Bilirubin = negative
Urobilinogen = negative
Blood = negative
WBC = 0-1/hpf
RBC = 3-5/hpf
Epithelial cells/hpf = occasional
Bacteria = negative
Casts = negative
Crystals = negative
Sperm = negative
Fat = negative

41. Collect stool for fecal flotation.

41. Negative.

42. Perform a skin scraping.

42. No mites seen.

43. Pluck some hairs for fungal culture.

43. No fungal growth.

44. Collect blood for a reticulocyte count.

44. Reticulocytes = 0%.

45. Collect blood for a serum thyroid hormone assay.

45. T_4 = 1.0 µg/dl.

Go to Section D

Section D:

Considering the information you have gained so far, what further diagnostic tests/therapeutic measures would you like to perform? (*Choose only the tests you believe relevant to managing the case at this point.*)

46. Collect blood for fasting and postprandial serum bile acids determination.

46. Fasting serum bile acids = 5 mmol/L; postprandial serum bile acids = 6 mmol/L.

47. Collect blood before and after ACTH administration for serum cortisol analysis.

47. Pre-ACTH cortisol = 3.5 µg/dl; Post-ACTH cortisol = 14.2 µg/dl.

48. Collect blood before and at 3 and 8 hours after administration of 0.015 mg/kg dexamethasone IV for serum cortisol analysis.

48. Pre-dexamethasone cortisol = 3.2 µg/dl; 3-hour post-dexamethasone cortisol = 1.0 µg/dl; 8-hour post-dexamethasone cortisol = 0.8 µg/dl.

49. Sedate the dog and perform several biopsies of affected and nonaffected skin.

49. Orthokeratotic hyperkeratosis with dermal atrophy and melanosis; consistent with an endocrine disorder.

50. Perform an electrocardiogram.

50. No abnormal findings.

51. Refer the dog to a specialist for thyroid gland nuclear imaging.

51. Scheduled.

52. Sedate the dog and collect bone marrow from the wing of the ilium.

52. Normal.

53. Refer the dog to a specialist for computerized tomogram of the pituitary gland.

53. Normal.

54. Collect blood before and 3 and 8 hours after administration of 0.15 mg/kg dexamethasone IV for serum cortisol analysis.

54. Results pending.

55. Ultrasound the abdomen.

55. No abnormal findings other than mild hepatomegaly.

56. Collect blood for a plasma endogenous ACTH assay.

56. Results pending.

57. Collect blood before and 6 hours after administration of TSH for serum thyroid hormone analysis.

57. Pre-TSH T_4 = 1.0 µg/dl; post-TSH T_4 = 1.0 µg/dl.

58. Anesthetize the dog and perform an ultrasound-guided liver biopsy.

58. Normal liver with mild lipid infiltrates.

Go to Section E

Section E:

Which course of action would you take? *(Choose only one.)*

59. Prescribe cephalexin and schedule a recheck examination in 2 weeks.

59. End of problem.

60. Prescribe an immunosuppressive dose of prednisone to be tapered over the next 3 months to alternate day therapy.

60. End of problem.

61. Prescribe o,p'-DDD (mitotane) at a dose of 25 mg/kg daily for 10 days; schedule a recheck examination in 10 days.

61. End of problem.

62. Prescribe thyroid hormone replacement therapy and schedule a recheck examination in 1 month.

62. End of problem.

63. Refer the dog to a specialist for further workup.

63. End of problem.

64. Prescribe a protein-restricted diet and give the owners a poor prognosis.

64. End of problem.

END OF PROBLEM

PARAMETER	UNITS	DOG*	CAT*	COCKATIEL†	PARROT†	BUDGIE†	IGUANA‡	PYTHON‡	FERRET§
CBC									
Hematocrit	%	37-55	25-45	36-49	37-50	38-48	38-52	25-40	46-57
Hemoglobin	g/dL	12.0-18	8.0-15	11.0-16	11-17.5	12.0-16	11.7-18.6		15.2-17.7
WBC	$\times 10^3$/uL	6.0-17	5.5-19.5	5.0-10.0	6.0-11	3.0-8.5	1.7-15	6.0-12	5.6-10.8
Neutrophils	$\times 10^3$/uL	3.0-11.5	2.5-12.5					0-2.4	0.6-7
Bands	$\times 10^3$/uL	0-0.3	0-0.3					0	0-0.2
Lymphocytes	$\times 10^3$/uL	1-4.8	1.5-7	1-4.5	1.2-5	0.7-4	0.6-9	0.6-7.2	1.4-5.6
Monocytes	$\times 10^3$/uL	0.1-1.4	0-0.8	0-0.2	0-0.3	0-0.2	0.2-5	0-0.4	0-0.4
Eosinophils	$\times 10^3$/uL	0.1-1.2	0-1.5	0-0.2	0-0.1	0-0.2	0-0.2	0-0.4	0-0.5
Basophils	$\times 10^3$/uL	rare	rare	0-0.1	0-0.1	0-0.1	0-1.5	0-1.2	0-0.2
Heterophils	$\times 10^3$/uL			2.7-8.0	3.3-8.8	1.5-6.5	0.1-8	0.7-7.2	
Platelets	$\times 10^3$/uL	200-500	200-500						300-700
MCV	fl	60-72	39-50	90-200	85-200	90-200			54-61
MCHC	g/dL	34-38	33-37	22-33	22-32	23-30			32-33
MCH	pg	22-27	13-18	28-55	28-55	25-60			17-20
Serum Chemistry Profile									
Glucose	mg/dL	65-122	67-124	200-445	190-345	190-390	150-280	10.0-60	90-125
BUN	mg/dL	7.0-28	17-32	2.9-5	3.1-5.3		6.0-15	1.0-10	12.0-43
Creatinine	mg/dL	0.6-1.5	0.6-2	0.1-0.4	0.1-0.4	0.1-0.4	0.1-0.7	0.1-0.3	0.2-0.6
Albumin	g/dL	2.7-4.5	2.3-3.9	0.7-1.8	1.9-3.5		1.0-1.6		3.3-4.1
Total protein	g/dL	5.4-7.4	5.9-8.1	3.2-5.6			2.8-6.9	5.0-8	5.3-7.2
ALT	IU/L	10-120	30-100	5.0-11	5.0-11				82-289
GGT	IU/L	0-6.0	0-1	1.0-30	1.0-12	1.0-10			
SAP	IU/L	18-141	6-106	20-250	15-150	10.0-80			30-120
Amylase	IU/L	50-1250	600-1200		205-510				
Cholesterol	mg/dL	130-300	60-220	140-360	180-305	145-275	110-341		119-209
Sodium	meq/L	145-158	146-160	140-153	125-155	139-165	140-183	130-152	146-160
Potassium	meq/L	4.1-5.5	3.7-5.4	2.4-4.6	3.0-4.5	2.2-3.9	1.3-5.2	3.0-5.7	4.3-5.3
Chloride	meq/L	106-127	112-129				102-125		102-121
Calcium	mg/dL	9-11.2	8.5-11	8.0-13	8.5-14	6.5-11	9.0-25.1	10.0-22	8.6-10.5
Phosphorus	mg/dL	2.8-6.1	3.3-7.8	3.2-4.8	3.1-5.5	3.0-5.2	3.5-9.8		5.6-8.7
T. Bilirubin	mg/dL	0-0.4	0-0.3				0.4-1.0		0-0.1

*Normal values established at Colorado State University.

†*Avian Medicine and Surgery*, Altman RB, Clubb SL, Dorrestien GM, and Quesenberry K, editors, Philadelphia, 1997, WB Saunders.

‡Rosskopf WJ, Woerpel RW, and Yanoff S: Normal hemogram and blood chemistry values for boa constrictors and pythons, *Vet Med* 77:822, 1982.

§*Ferrets, rabbits and rodents, clinical medicine and surgery*. Hillyer EV, Quesenberry KE, editors, Philadelphia, 1997, WB Saunders.

continued

PARAMETER	UNITS	DOG*	CAT*	COCKATIEL†	PARROT†	BUDGIE†	IGUANA‡	PYTHON‡	FERRET§
Serum Chemistry Profile—cont'd									
Total CO_2	mmol/L	14-27	17-24	13-25	13-26	14-25			16-28
Lipase	IU/L	30-560	3-125	30-280	35-225				
Preprandial bile acids	µmol/L	<10	<10	20-85	18-60	15-70			
Postprandial bile acids	µmol/L	<15	<15						
Urinalysis									
Color		yellow	yellow						
Character		clear to slightly cloudy							
Specific gravity		1.001-1.050	1.001-1.060						
pH		5.5-7	5.5-7						
Protein		0-2+	0-2+						
Glucose		neg	neg						
Ketones		neg	neg						
Bilirubin		0-2+	neg						
Urobilinogen	ehrlich units	0.1-1	0.1-1						
Blood		neg	neg						
WBC	per hpf	0-5	0-5						
RBC	per hpf	0-5	0-5						
Epithelial cells	per hpf	0-5	0-5						
Casts	per hpf	0-2	0-2						
Crystals	per hpf	variable	variable						
Bacteria	per hpf	none	none						
Endocrine									
T4	µg/dL	1.43-4	1.2-4.8				1.5-4.6		1.5-3.6||
Free T4	ng/dL	0.35-1.4	0.65-1.5						0.5-1.2
T3	ng/dL	0.8-1.5	0.7-1.1						1.5-3.6
Pre-TSH T4	µg/dL	1.43-4	1.2-4.8						2.3-4.5
Post-TSH T4	µg/dL	double baseline	double baseline						0.2-2.2
Resting cortisol	µg/dL	1-6.2	1-6.2						3.1-7.2
Post-ACTH cortisol	µg/dL	10.5-20	10.5-20						<0.3
3-hour post-dexamethasone cortisol	µg/dL	<1	<1						
8-hour post-dexamethasone cortisol	µg/dL	<1	<1						
Urine cortisol: creatinine ratio		<1	<1						
Endogenous ACTH	pg/mL	20-80	20-80						
Parathyroid hormone	pmol/L	1.0-8							

||Heard DJ, Collins B, Chen DL et al: Thyroid and adrenal function tests in adult male ferrets, *Am J Vet Res* 51:32, 1990.

As in the CCT, the answer choices in this book are "weighted" with regard to point value. Some answer choices are "clearly indicated" (essential in resolving the case), some are "clearly contraindicated " (must be avoided in managing the case), and some are "neutral" (neither indicated nor contraindicated). Answer choices that are clearly indicated are signified by a "+." Choices that are clearly contraindicated are signified by a "–." Choices that are neither indicated nor contraindicated are signified by a "0."

PROBLEM 1 Answer Key

1. +	20. +	39. +
2. +	21. +	40. +
3. +	22. −	41. 0
4. +	23. +	42. −
5. 0	24. +	43. −
6. +	25. −	44. +
7. 0	26. −	45. −
8. +	27. 0	46. −
9. 0	28. 0	47. −
10. +	29. −	48. +
11. +	30. +	49. −
12. +	31. −	50. −
13. +	32. 0	51. −
14. −	33. −	52. −
15. −	34. −	53. +
16. +	35. −	54. −
17. 0	36. −	55. −
18. +	37. −	56. −
19. +	38. −	57. −

+ = clearly indicated   − = contraindicated   0 = neutral

Total Positive Responses _____

Total Neutral Responses _____

Total Negative Responses _____

RECOMMENDED READING

Joyner KL: Avian reproductive emergency—medical management, *Vet Med Report* 2:246-249, 1990.

Martin HD: Avian reproductive emergency—surgical management, *Vet Med Report* 2:250-253, 1990.

Ritchie, Harrison, and Harrison: *Avian medicine: principles and application,* Lake Worth, Fla, 1994, Wingers Publishing, Inc., Chapters 3 (Nutrition), 8 (Making distinctions in the physical exam), and 29 (Theriogenology).

Rosskopf WJ, Woerpel R, editors: Veterinary clinics of North America (small animal practice), *Avian Pet Med* 21:6, 1991.

Snyder RL, Terry J: Avian nutrition. In Fowler M, editor: *Zoo and wild animal medicine,* ed 2, Philadelphia, 1986, WB Saunders.

PROBLEM 2 Answer Key

1. −	31. +	61. −
2. −	32. −	62. −
3. 0	33. −	63. −
4. +	34. −	64. −
5. −	35. −	65. −
6. −	36. 0	66. 0
7. +	37. +	67. 0
8. +	38. +	68. −
9. +	39. +	69. −
10. +	40. −	70. −
11. +	41. 0	71. −
12. +	42. 0	72. −
13. +	43. 0	73. +
14. +	44. +	74. +
15. 0	45. +	75. −
16. +	46. +	76. −
17. +	47. +	77. −
18. +	48. +	78. −
19. 0	49. −	79. −
20. 0	50. −	80. +
21. 0	51. −	81. −
22. 0	52. −	82. −
23. +	53. +	83. +
24. 0	54. +	84. +
25. +	55. +	85. −
26. +	56. +	86. −
27. −	57. +	87. −
28. +	58. 0	88. −
29. +	59. 0	89. −
30. +	60. +	

+ = clearly indicated   − = contraindicated   0 = neutral

Total Positive Responses _____

Total Neutral Responses _____

Total Negative Responses _____

RECOMMENDED READING

Fudge A, editor: Chlamydiosis. In *Seminars in avian and exotic pet medicine,* Philadelphia, 1993, vol 24(4), WB Saunders.

Ritchie BW, Harrison GJ, Harrison LR: *Avian medicine: principles and application,* Lake Worth, Fla., 1994, Wingers Publishing, Inc., Chapters 3 (Nutrition), 8 (Making distinctions in the physical exam), and 34 (Chlamydia).

Rosskopf WJ, Woerpel R, editors: Veterinary clinics of North America (small animal practice), *Avian Pet Med* 21:6, Nov. 1991.

PROBLEM 3 Answer Key

1. +	24. –	47. –
2. +	25. +	48. 0
3. +	26. +	49. 0
4. +	27. –	50. 0
5. +	28. –	51. –
6. 0	29. –	52. –
7. +	30. +	53. 0
8. 0	31. –	54. –
9. 0	32. –	55. –
10. 0	33. –	56. –
11. +	34. 0	57. –
12. +	35. 0	58. –
13. 0	36. –	59. –
14. +	37. –	60. –
15. +	38. –	61. –
16. +	39. 0	62. +
17. +	40. –	63. –
18. –	41. 0	64. –
19. +	42. +	65. –
20. –	43. –	66. –
21. +	44. –	67. –
22. +	45. –	68. –
23. –	46. –	

+ = clearly indicated   – = contraindicated   0 = neutral

Total Positive Responses _____

Total Neutral Responses _____

Total Negative Responses _____

RECOMMENDED READING

Ritchie BW, Harrison GJ, Harrison LR: *Avian medicine: principles and application,* Lake Worth, Fla., 1994, Wingers Publishing, Inc., Chapters 8 (Making distinctions in the physical exam) and 36 (Parasites).

Rosskopf WJ and Woerpel R, editors: Veterinary clinics of North America (small animal practice), *Avian Pet Med* 21:6, Nov. 1991.

PROBLEM 4 Answer Key

1. +	20. +	39. –
2. 0	21. –	40. –
3. +	22. –	41. +
4. +	23. –	42. –
5. +	24. –	43. +
6. +	25. +	44. –
7. 0	26. +	45. –
8. +	27. +	46. –
9. +	28. –	47. –
10. +	29. 0	48. –
11. 0	30. 0	49. –
12. 0	31. –	50. –
13. +	32. –	51. –
14. +	33. –	52. –
15. +	34. –	53. –
16. +	35. –	54. –
17. +	36. –	55. +
18. –	37. –	56. –
19. +	38. –	57. –

+ = clearly indicated   – = contraindicated   0 = neutral

Total Positive Responses _____

Total Neutral Responses _____

Total Negative Responses _____

RECOMMENDED READING

Ritchie BW, Harrison GJ, Harrison LR: *Avian medicine: principles and application,* Lake Worth, Fla., 1994, Wingers Publishing, Inc., Chapters 1 (The avian patient), 2 (The avian flock), 6 (Future preventative medicine), and 32 (Viruses).

Ritchie BW, editor: *Avian viruses—function and control,* Lake Worth, Fla., 1995, Wingers Publishing, Inc., Chapter 6 (Papovaviridae).

Ritchie BW et al: *A Polyomavirus overview and evaluation of an experimental polyomavirus vaccine.* Proceedings of the AAV Annual Conference, 1992, pp. 1 - 4.

Ritchie BW et al: Polyomavirus infection in adult psittacine birds, *J Assoc Avian Vet* 5:147-153, 1991.

PROBLEM 5 Answer Key

1. +	25. +	49. −
2. 0	26. −	50. −
3. +	27. 0	51. −
4. +	28. +	52. −
5. +	29. +	53. −
6. +	30. −	54. +
7. −	31. 0	55. −
8. +	32. −	56. −
9. 0	33. −	57. −
10. 0	34. +	58. −
11. 0	35. −	59. −
12. +	36. −	60. +
13. 0	37. −	61. −
14. −	38. +	62. −
15. +	39. +	63. −
16. 0	40. +	64. −
17. 0	41. −	65. −
18. 0	42. −	66. +
19. +	43. −	67. −
20. +	44. −	68. −
21. 0	45. +	69. −
22. 0	46. 0	70. −
23. +	47. 0	71. −
24. 0	48. −	

+ = clearly indicated   − = contraindicated   0 = neutral

Total Positive Responses _____

Total Neutral Responses _____

Total Negative Responses _____

PROBLEM 6 Answer Key

1. 0	24. +	47. −
2. 0	25. +	48. −
3. 0	26. −	49. −
4. +	27. +	50. −
5. +	28. +	51. +
6. +	29. +	52. −
7. 0	30. −	53. −
8. +	31. +	54. −
9. +	32. −	55. −
10. +	33. −	56. −
11. +	34. +	57. −
12. +	35. 0	58. +
13. 0	36. −	59. +
14. −	37. −	60. −
15. +	38. −	61. −
16. +	39. −	62. −
17. +	40. −	63. −
18. +	41. −	64. +
19. +	42. −	65. −
20. +	43. −	66. −
21. 0	44. −	67. −
22. 0	45. +	68. −
23. +	46. 0	

+ = clearly indicated   − = contraindicated   0 = neutral

Total Positive Responses _____

Total Neutral Responses _____

Total Negative Responses _____

RECOMMENDED READING

Harkness JE, Wagner JE: *The biology and medicine of rabbits and rodents,* ed 3, Philadelphia, 1989, Lea and Febiger. (The fourth edition is now available.)

Manning PJ et al: *The biology of the laboratory rabbit,* ed 2, San Diego, 1994, Academic Press.

Quesenberry KE, Hillyer EV, editors: *Veterinary clinics of North America, exotic pet medicine 1,* Vol 23(6), Philadelphia, Nov. 1993, WB Saunders.

Quesenberry KE, Hillyer EV, editors: *Veterinary clinics of North America, exotic pet medicine 2,* Vol 23(1), Philadelphia, Jan. 1994, WB Saunders.

Wagner JE, Manning PJ: *The biology of the guinea pig,* San Diego, 1976, Academic Press.

PROBLEM 7 Answer Key

1. 0	22. –	42. 0
2. +	23. +	43. 0
3. +	24. +	44. 0
4. –	25. –	45. +
5. 0	26. –	46. –
6. +	27. +	47. 0
7. 0	28. 0	48. 0
8. +	29. –	49. –
9. +	30. +	50. –
10. +	31. +	51. –
11. 0	32. +	52. –
12. –	33. +	53. –
13. +	34. 0	54. –
14. 0	35. –	55. +
15. +	36. 0	56. –
16. +	37. –	57. –
17. 0	38. 0	58. –
18. +	39. +	59. +
19. –	40. –	60. –
20. +	41. 0	61. –
21. +		

+ = clearly indicated   – = contraindicated   0 = neutral

Total Positive Responses _____

Total Neutral Responses _____

Total Negative Responses _____

RECOMMENDED READING

Broussard JD, Peterson ME, Fox PR: Changes in clinical and laboratory findings in cats with hyperthyroidism from 1983 to 1993, *JAVMA* 206(3):302-305, 1995.

Feldman EC, Nelson RW: *Canine and feline endocrinology and reproduction,* Philadelphia, 1987, Saunders.

Graves TK, Peterson ME: Diagnostic tests for feline hyperthyroidism, *Vet Clin North Am (Small Anim Pract)* 24(3):567-576, 1994.

PROBLEM 8 Answer Key

1. 0	23. +	45. +
2. +	24. –	46. –
3. +	25. 0	47. –
4. +	26. +	48. –
5. 0	27. +	49. +
6. +	28. +	50. –
7. +	29. 0	51. +
8. +	30. 0	52. –
9. +	31. –	53. –
10. –	32. –	54. –
11. +	33. +	55. –
12. +	34. –	56. –
13. 0	35. –	57. 0
14. +	36. +	58. +
15. +	37. +	59. –
16. 0	38. +	60. –
17. 0	39. 0	61. –
18. +	40. 0	62. –
19. +	41. –	63. –
20. 0	42. +	64. +
21. +	43. 0	65. –
22. 0	44. 0	66. –

+ = clearly indicated   – = contraindicated   0 = neutral

Total Positive Responses _____

Total Neutral Responses _____

Total Negative Responses _____

RECOMMENDED READING

Feldman EC, Nelson RW: *Canine and feline endocrinology and reproduction,* Philadelphia, 1987, WB Saunders.

Kintzer PP, Peterson ME: In Bonagura, editor: *Kirk's current veterinary therapy XII, small animal practice,* Philadelphia, 1995, WB Saunders.

PROBLEM 9 Answer Key

1. 0	25. 0	49. +
2. +	26. 0	50. +
3. +	27. 0	51. +
4. +	28. +	52. −
5. +	29. −	53. −
6. +	30. −	54. −
7. +	31. +	55. 0
8. +	32. +	56. −
9. +	33. +	57. −
10. 0	34. 0	58. −
11. 0	35. 0	59. +
12. 0	36. −	60. −
13. +	37. +	61. −
14. 0	38. −	62. −
15. 0	39. −	63. +
16. −	40. +	64. −
17. +	41. −	65. −
18. +	42. −	66. +
19. −	43. 0	67. −
20. 0	44. 0	68. −
21. +	45. −	69. −
22. +	46. −	70. −
23. +	47. −	71. −
24. 0	48. −	72. +

+ = clearly indicated   − = contraindicated   0 = neutral

Total Positive Responses _____

Total Neutral Responses _____

Total Negative Responses _____

RECOMMENDED READING

Cowgill LD: In Bonagura JD, editor: *Kirk's current veterinary therapy XII, small animal practice,* Philadelphia, 1995, WB Saunders.

Finco DR, Brown SA: In Bonagura JD, editor: *Kirk's current veterinary therapy XII, small animal practice,* Philadelphia, 1995, WB Saunders.

Lulich JP et al: Feline renal failure: questions, answers, questions, *Compend Cont Educ* 14(2):127-152, 1992.

Polzin DJ et al: In Ettinger SJ and Feldman EC, editors: *Textbook of veterinary internal medicine,* Philadelphia, 1995, WB Saunders.

Ross LA: Hypertension and chronic renal failure, *Sem in Vet Med and Surg (Small Anim)* 7(3):221-226, 1992.

PROBLEM 10 Answer Key

1. +	24. +	47. 0
2. +	25. −	48. −
3. +	26. −	49. +
4. −	27. +	50. 0
5. +	28. +	51. 0
6. +	29. 0	52. −
7. +	30. +	53. −
8. +	31. +	54. −
9. +	32. +	55. +
10. −	33. +	56. +
11. +	34. −	57. 0
12. +	35. +	58. −
13. −	36. +	59. −
14. +	37. +	60. 0
15. +	38. −	61. 0
16. 0	39. 0	62. −
17. +	40. 0	63. −
18. 0	41. +	64. +
19. +	42. −	65. −
20. +	43. −	66. −
21. +	44. −	67. −
22. +	45. 0	68. −
23. +	46. +	69. −

+ = clearly indicated   − = contraindicated   0 = neutral

Total Positive Responses _____

Total Neutral Responses _____

Total Negative Responses _____

RECOMMENDED READING

Grauer GF: Glomerulonephritis, *Sem in Vet Med and Surg (Small Anim)* 7(3):187-197, 1992.

Grauer GF, DiBartola SP: In Ettinger SJ, Feldman EC, editors: *Textbook of veterinary internal medicine,* Philadelphia, 1995, WB Saunders.

Knight DH: In Bonagura JD, editor: *Kirk's current veterinary therapy XII, small animal practice,* Philadelphia, 1995, WB Saunders

Vaden SL, Grauer GF: In Kirk RW, editor: *Current veterinary therapy XI, small animal practice,* Philadelphia, 1992, WB Saunders.

PROBLEM 11 Answer Key

1. +	20. 0	39. +
2. +	21. 0	40. +
3. +	22. +	41. +
4. +	23. +	42. +
5. +	24. –	43. +
6. 0	25. +	44. +
7. 0	26. 0	45. +
8. 0	27. +	46. –
9. +	28. 0	47. 0
10. 0	29. +	48. +
11. 0	30. +	49. +
12. +	31. +	50. +
13. +	32. +	51. –
14. 0	33. 0	52. –
15. +	34. –	53. –
16. +	35. –	54. +
17. +	36. –	55. –
18. +	37. –	56. –
19. +	38. –	57. –

+ = clearly indicated   – = contraindicated   0 = neutral

Total Positive Responses _____

Total Neutral Responses _____

Total Negative Responses _____

RECOMMENDED READING

Bauer T, Woodfield JA: In Ettinger SJ, Feldman EC, editors: *Textbook of veterinary internal medicine,* ed 4, Philadelphia, 1995, WB Saunders, pp. 824-825.

Roudebush P: In Greene CE, editor: *Infectious diseases of the dog and cat,* Philadelphia, 1990, WB Saunders, pp. 122-123.

Vaden SL, Papich MG: In Bonagura JD, editor: *Kirk's current veterinary therapy XII, small animal practice,* Philadelphia, 1995, WB Saunders, pp. 276-280.

PROBLEM 12 Answer Key

1. +	20. +	39. –
2. +	21. 0	40. –
3. +	22. 0	41. +
4. +	23. –	42. –
5. 0	24. +	43. +
6. +	25. –	44. +
7. 0	26. –	45. 0
8. 0	27. –	46. –
9. +	28. 0	47. –
10. 0	29. 0	48. +
11. 0	30. 0	49. +
12. +	31. +	50. –
13. +	32. +	51. –
14. +	33. –	52. +
15. +	34. +	53. +
16. +	35. 0	54. –
17. 0	36. +	55. –
18. +	37. +	56. –
19. +	38. 0	

+ = clearly indicated   – = contraindicated   0 = neutral

Total Positive Responses _____

Total Neutral Responses _____

Total Negative Responses _____

RECOMMENDED READING

Barsanti JA, Jeffery KL: In Greene CE, editor: *Infectious diseases of the dog and cat,* Philadelphia, 1990, WB Saunders, pp. 707-710.

Legendre A: In Bonagura JD, editor: *Kirk's current veterinary therapy XII small animal practice,* Philadelphia, 1995, WB Saunders, pp. 327-331.

Wolf AM, Troy GC: In Ettinger SJ, Feldman EC, editors: *Textbook of veterinary internal medicine,* ed 4, Philadelphia, 1995, WB Saunders, pp. 453-455.

PROBLEM 13 Answer Key

1. +	20. +	38. –
2. +	21. +	39. –
3. +	22. +	40. –
4. +	23. 0	41. –
5. +	24. +	42. –
6. +	25. 0	43. –
7. 0	26. –	44. –
8. +	27. –	45. +
9. +	28. +	46. 0
10. 0	29. +	47. –
11. 0	30. +	48. +
12. +	31. +	49. +
13. +	32. –	50. +
14. +	33. +	51. –
15. 0	34. +	52. –
16. +	35. 0	53. –
17. +	36. +	54. –
18. +	37. +	55. –
19. +		

+ = clearly indicated   – = contraindicated   0 = neutral

Total Positive Responses _____

Total Neutral Responses _____

Total Negative Responses _____

RECOMMENDED READING

Barsanti JA, Jeffery KL: In Greene CE, editor: *Infectious diseases of the dog and cat,* Philadelphia, 1990, WB Saunders, pp. 696-706.

Legendre A: In Bonagura JD, editor: *Kirk's current veterinary therapy XII small animal practice,* Philadelphia, 1995, WB Saunders, pp. 327-331.

Wolf AM, Troy GC: In Ettinger SJ, Feldman EC, editors: *Textbook of veterinary internal medicine,* ed 4, Philadelphia, 1995, WB Saunders, pp. 444-448.

PROBLEM 14 Answer Key

1. +	16. +	31. –
2. +	17. +	32. –
3. +	18. 0	33. 0
4. 0	19. +	34. –
5. +	20. +	35. –
6. +	21. 0	36. –
7. +	22. +	37. –
8. +	23. +	38. –
9. +	24. –	39. –
10. –	25. –	40. –
11. +	26. 0	41. +
12. +	27. 0	42. +
13. –	28. 0	43. –
14. +	29. 0	44. –
15. +	30. –	45. –

+ = clearly indicated   – = contraindicated   0 = neutral

Total Positive Responses _____

Total Neutral Responses _____

Total Negative Responses _____

RECOMMENDED READING

Draper CS et al: Patterns of oral bacterial infection in captive snakes, *JAVMA* 179:1223, 1981.

Hilf M et al: A prospective study of upper airway flora in healthy boid snakes and snakes with pneumonia, *J Zoo and Wildlife Med* 21:318, 1990.

Rosskopf WJ et al: Normal hemogram and blood chemistry values for boa constrictors and pythons, *Vet Med* 77:822, May 1982.

PROBLEM 15 Answer Key

1. +	20. 0	39. −
2. +	21. 0	40. 0
3. +	22. −	41. +
4. +	23. +	42. −
5. +	24. +	43. −
6. +	25. 0	44. 0
7. +	26. 0	45. −
8. +	27. 0	46. −
9. +	28. +	47. −
10. 0	29. +	48. +
11. +	30. −	49. +
12. 0	31. −	50. +
13. +	32. −	51. −
14. +	33. 0	52. +
15. +	34. −	53. −
16. +	35. −	54. +
17. 0	36. −	55. +
18. 0	37. +	56. +
19. 0	38. −	57. +

+ = clearly indicated   − = contraindicated   0 = neutral

Total Positive Responses _____

Total Neutral Responses _____

Total Negative Responses _____

RECOMMENDED READING

Bayer TH: Metabolic bone disease. In Mader DR, editor: *Reptile medicine and surgery,* Philadelphia, 1996, WB Saunders.

PROBLEM 16 Answer Key

1. +	17. +	33. 0
2. +	18. +	34. −
3. +	19. +	35. −
4. +	20. 0	36. −
5. 0	21. +	37. −
6. 0	22. +	38. −
7. 0	23. 0	39. 0
8. 0	24. +	40. −
9. +	25. +	41. +
10. +	26. −	42. −
11. −	27. +	43. 0
12. −	28. −	44. +
13. +	29. −	45. −
14. 0	30. −	46. −
15. +	31. −	47. 0
16. +	32. +	48. −

+ = clearly indicated   − = contraindicated   0 = neutral

Total Positive Responses _____

Total Neutral Responses _____

Total Negative Responses _____

RECOMMENDED READING

Brown SA: Adrenal and pancreatic neoplasia, *Proc NA Vet Conf* 7:725, 1993.

Gould WJ et al: Evaluation of urinary cortisol: creatinine ratios for diagnosis of hyperadrenocorticism associated with adrenocortical tumors in ferrets, *JAVMA* 206:42, 1995.

Heard DJ et al: Thyroid and adrenal function tests in adult male ferrets, *Am J Vet Res* 51:32, 1990.

Jenkins JR, Brown SA: Alopecia. In *Practitioner's guide to rabbits and ferrets,* 1993, Lakewood, Colo., American Animal Hospital Association.

Rosenthal K: Ferrets, *Vet Clin North Am* 24:16, 1994.

Rosenthal K et al: Hyperadrenocorticism associated with adrenocortical tumor or nodular hyperplasia of the adrenal glands in ferrets. 50 cases (1987-1991), *JAVMA* 203:271, 1993.

PROBLEM 17 Answer Key

1. +	19. +	37. −
2. +	20. +	38. +
3. 0	21. +	39. −
4. 0	22. +	40. +
5. +	23. +	41. −
6. +	24. 0	42. −
7. 0	25. 0	43. +
8. 0	26. −	44. −
9. 0	27. −	45. −
10. 0	28. −	46. −
11. +	29. +	47. −
12. 0	30. 0	48. +
13. 0	31. 0	49. −
14. +	32. +	50. −
15. +	33. 0	51. 0
16. +	34. −	52. +
17. +	35. 0	53. −
18. +	36. −	54. −

+ = clearly indicated   − = contraindicated   0 = neutral

Total Positive Responses _____

Total Neutral Responses _____

Total Negative Responses _____

RECOMMENDED READING

Ehrhart N et al: Insulin secreting tumors in the ferret: 20 cases, *JAVMA* 209(10):1737, 1996.

Elie MS, Zerbe CA: Insulinoma in dogs, cats, and ferrets, *Comp Cont Educ* 17:51, 1995.

Hillyer EV, Brown SA: Ferrets. In Birchard SJ and Sherding RG, editors: *Saunders manual of small animal practice,* 1994, Philadelphia, WB Saunders.

Mann FA et al: Reference intervals for insulin concentrations and insulin:glucose ratios in the serum of ferrets, *J Sm Exotic An Med* 2:79, 1993.

Marini RP et al: Functional islet cell tumor in six ferrets, *JAVMA* 202:430, 1993.

Rosenthal K: Ferret insulinoma, *Proc N AM Vet Conf* 9:581, 1995.

PROBLEM 18 Answer Key

1. +	22. 0	43. −
2. +	23. 0	44. +
3. +	24. +	45. −
4. +	25. 0	46. −
5. +	26. 0	47. +
6. +	27. 0	48. −
7. 0	28. 0	49. −
8. 0	29. 0	50. −
9. 0	30. −	51. +
10. 0	31. −	52. −
11. 0	32. −	53. +
12. 0	33. −	54. 0
13. 0	34. −	55. −
14. 0	35. +	56. −
15. +	36. −	57. −
16. +	37. +	58. −
17. +	38. +	59. −
18. +	39. +	60. +
19. 0	40. −	61. −
20. 0	41. −	62. −
21. 0	42. −	

+ = clearly indicated   − = contraindicated   0 = neutral

Total Positive Responses _____

Total Neutral Responses _____

Total Negative Responses _____

RECOMMENDED READING

Fossum TW: Chylothorax, recent advances and new perspectives, *Vet Med Report* 1:300, 1989.

Fossum TW, Birchard SJ, Jacobs RM: Chylothorax in 34 dogs, *JAVMA* 188:1315, 1986.

Fossum TW, Jacobs RM, Birchard SJ: Evaluation of cholesterol and triglyceride concentrations in differentiating chylous and nonchylous pleural effusions in dogs and cats, *JAVMA* 188:49, 1986.

PROBLEM 19 Answer Key

1. +	23. 0	44. –
2. +	24. 0	45. –
3. +	25. +	46. –
4. +	26. 0	47. +
5. 0	27. 0	48. –
6. +	28. +	49. +
7. +	29. 0	50. –
8. +	30. 0	51. 0
9. 0	31. 0	52. +
10. 0	32. +	53. 0
11. 0	33. +	54. –
12. 0	34. 0	55. 0
13. 0	35. 0	56. –
14. 0	36. 0	57. –
15. 0	37. –	58. –
16. 0	38. –	59. –
17. +	39. –	60. –
18. +	40. –	61. –
19. 0	41. +	62. –
20. 0	42. –	63. –
21. 0	43. –	64. +
22. 0		

+ = clearly indicated   – = contraindicated   0 = neutral

Total Positive Responses _____

Total Neutral Responses _____

Total Negative Responses _____

RECOMMENDED READING

Medleau L, Barsanti JA: Cryptococcosis. In Greene CE, editor: *Infectious diseases of the dog and cat,* Philadelphia, 1990, WB Saunders.

PROBLEM 20 Answer Key

1. +	22. +	43. 0
2. +	23. 0	44. –
3. +	24. 0	45. –
4. +	25. 0	46. –
5. 0	26. 0	47. –
6. +	27. +	48. –
7. +	28. 0	49. –
8. +	29. 0	50. –
9. 0	30. +	51. –
10. +	31. 0	52. 0
11. 0	32. 0	53. +
12. 0	33. +	54. –
13. 0	34. –	55. –
14. +	35. –	56. –
15. 0	36. –	57. –
16. +	37. –	58. –
17. +	38. +	59. –
18. +	39. –	60. –
19. +	40. +	61. +
20. +	41. –	62. –
21. 0	42. –	

+ = clearly indicated   – = contraindicated   0 = neutral

Total Positive Responses _____

Total Neutral Responses _____

Total Negative Responses _____

RECOMMENDED READING

Atkins CE: Acquired valvular insufficiency. In Miller MS, Tilley LP, editors: *Manual of canine and feline cardiology,* ed 2, Philadelphia, 1995, WB Saunders.

Keene BW, Rush JE: Therapy of heart failure. In Ettinger SJ, editor: *Textbook of veterinary internal medicine,* ed 3, Philadelphia, 1989, WB Saunders.

PROBLEM 21 Answer Key

1. +	20. +	38. −
2. +	21. 0	39. +
3. +	22. 0	40. 0
4. +	23. 0	41. −
5. 0	24. 0	42. +
6. +	25. +	43. −
7. +	26. 0	44. −
8. +	27. +	45. −
9. 0	28. 0	46. −
10. 0	29. 0	47. −
11. 0	30. 0	48. −
12. 0	31. 0	49. +
13. 0	32. 0	50. −
14. 0	33. 0	51. −
15. 0	34. 0	52. −
16. +	35. +	53. +
17. +	36. 0	54. −
18. +	37. +	55. −
19. +		

+ = clearly indicated   − = contraindicated   0 = neutral

Total Positive Responses _____

Total Neutral Responses _____

Total Negative Responses _____

RECOMMENDED READING

Pion PD, Kienle RD: Feline cardiomyopathy. In Miller MS and Tilley LP, editors: *Manual of canine and feline cardiology,* ed 2, Philadelphia, 1995, WB Saunders.

Pion PD, Kittleson MD: Therapy of feline aortic thromboembolism. In Kirk RW, editor: *Current veterinary therapy IX,* Philadelphia, 1989, WB Saunders.

PROBLEM 22 Answer Key

1. +	22. +	43. −
2. +	23. 0	44. −
3. +	24. +	45. −
4. +	25. 0	46. −
5. 0	26. 0	47. 0
6. +	27. 0	48. −
7. +	28. 0	49. −
8. +	29. 0	50. −
9. +	30. +	51. −
10. +	31. +	52. −
11. 0	32. +	53. +
12. 0	33. −	54. 0
13. +	34. +	55. +
14. 0	35. −	56. −
15. 0	36. +	57. −
16. +	37. −	58. −
17. +	38. −	59. −
18. +	39. +	60. −
19. 0	40. 0	61. +
20. 0	41. −	62. −
21. +	42. 0	63. −

+ = clearly indicated   − = contraindicated   0 = neutral

Total Positive Responses _____

Total Neutral Responses _____

Total Negative Responses _____

RECOMMENDED READING

Hall JA, Macy DW, Husted PW: Acute canine pancreatitis, *Comp Cont Educ* 10:403, 1988.

PROBLEM 23 Answer Key

1. +	20. 0	38. 0
2. +	21. 0	39. −
3. +	22. +	40. +
4. 0	23. 0	41. −
5. 0	24. 0	42. −
6. 0	25. +	43. −
7. 0	26. 0	44. +
8. +	27. 0	45. −
9. 0	28. +	46. −
10. +	29. 0	47. −
11. 0	30. +	48. −
12. 0	31. 0	49. −
13. +	32. +	50. −
14. +	33. +	51. −
15. 0	34. +	52. −
16. 0	35. 0	53. −
17. 0	36. 0	54. +
18. 0	37. −	55. −
19. 0		

+ = clearly indicated   − = contraindicated   0 = neutral

Total Positive Responses _____

Total Neutral Responses _____

Total Negative Responses _____

RECOMMENDED READING

Barlough JE, Stoddart CA: Feline coronaviral infections. In Greene CE, editor: *Infectious diseases of the dog and cat,* Philadelphia, 1990, WB Saunders.

Weiss RC: Feline infectious peritonitis virus: Advances in therapy and control. In August JR, editor: *Consultations in feline medicine 2,* Philadelphia, 1994, WB Saunders.

PROBLEM 24 Answer Key

1. +	22. +	43. 0
2. +	23. +	44. 0
3. +	24. +	45. −
4. +	25. 0	46. +
5. 0	26. 0	47. +
6. +	27. 0	48. 0
7. +	28. 0	49. 0
8. +	29. +	50. 0
9. +	30. +	51. +
10. +	31. +	52. −
11. +	32. +	53. +
12. +	33. +	54. −
13. 0	34. −	55. 0
14. 0	35. +	56. −
15. 0	36. +	57. −
16. 0	37. 0	58. +
17. 0	38. 0	59. −
18. 0	39. +	60. −
19. 0	40. +	61. −
20. 0	41. +	62. −
21. 0	42. 0	

+ = clearly indicated   − = contraindicated   0 = neutral

Total Positive Responses _____

Total Neutral Responses _____

Total Negative Responses _____

RECOMMENDED READING

Chew DS, Carothers MA: Hypercalcemia, *Vet Clin North Am* 19:265, 1989.

Meuten DJ, Armstrong PJ: Parathyroid disease and calcium metabolism. In Ettinger SJ, editor: *Textbook of veterinary internal medicine,* ed 3, Philadelphia, 1989, WB Saunders.

PROBLEM 25 Answer Key

1. +	22. 0	43. –
2. +	23. 0	44. –
3. +	24. 0	45. 0
4. +	25. 0	46. –
5. 0	26. 0	47. –
6. +	27. +	48. 0
7. +	28. 0	49. –
8. +	29. +	50. 0
9. 0	30. +	51. 0
10. 0	31. +	52. 0
11. 0	32. +	53. –
12. 0	33. 0	54. –
13. 0	34. –	55. –
14. 0	35. +	56. –
15. 0	36. +	57. +
16. 0	37. 0	58. –
17. 0	38. 0	59. –
18. 0	39. 0	60. –
19. 0	40. –	61. –
20. 0	41. +	62. –
21. +	42. 0	

+ = clearly indicated   – = contraindicated   0 = neutral

Total Positive Responses _____

Total Neutral Responses _____

Total Negative Responses _____

RECOMMENDED READING

Feldman EC, Nelson RW: Diabetes mellitus. In Feldman EC, Nelson RW, editors: *Canine and feline endocrinology and reproduction,* ed 2, Philadelphia, 1996, WB Saunders.

Nelson RW: Diabetes mellitus. In Birchard SJ, Sherding RG, editors: *Saunders manual of small animal practice,* Philadelphia, 1994, WB Saunders.

PROBLEM 26 Answer Key

1. +	22. 0	43. 0
2. +	23. +	44. 0
3. +	24. 0	45. +
4. +	25. 0	46. 0
5. 0	26. 0	47. –
6. +	27. +	48. –
7. +	28. 0	49. –
8. +	29. +	50. –
9. +	30. +	51. 0
10. +	31. +	52. –
11. 0	32. +	53. +
12. +	33. 0	54. +
13. 0	34. –	55. 0
14. +	35. 0	56. –
15. 0	36. +	57. –
16. 0	37. 0	58. –
17. 0	38. 0	59. +
18. 0	39. +	60. –
19. 0	40. 0	61. –
20. 0	41. –	62. –
21. 0	42. +	

+ = clearly indicated   – = contraindicated   0 = neutral

Total Positive Responses _____

Total Neutral Responses _____

Total Negative Responses _____

RECOMMENDED READING

Griffiths GL, Lumsden JH, Valli VEO: Hematologic and biochemical changes in dogs with portosystemic shunts, *J Am Animal Hosp Assoc* 17:705, 1981.

Johnson CA, Armstrong PJ, Hauptman JG: Congenital portosystemic shunts in dogs: 46 cases (1979-1986), *JAVMA* 191:1478, 1987.

Meyer DJ, Harvey JW: Hematologic changes associated with serum and hepatic iron alterations in dogs with congenital portosystemic vascular anomalies, *J Vet Internal Med* 8:55, 1994.

PROBLEM 27 Answer Key

1. +	23. 0	44. –
2. +	24. 0	45. 0
3. +	25. 0	46. –
4. +	26. 0	47. –
5. 0	27. 0	48. +
6. 0	28. +	49. +
7. +	29. +	50. –
8. 0	30. 0	51. –
9. 0	31. 0	52. –
10. 0	32. 0	53. –
11. 0	33. 0	54. –
12. 0	34. 0	55. –
13. 0	35. –	56. –
14. 0	36. 0	57. –
15. 0	37. 0	58. –
16. 0	38. +	59. –
17. 0	39. +	60. –
18. 0	40. +	61. –
19. 0	41. 0	62. +
20. +	42. 0	63. –
21. 0	43. 0	64. –
22. 0		

+ = clearly indicated   – = contraindicated   0 = neutral

Total Positive Responses _____

Total Neutral Responses _____

Total Negative Responses _____

RECOMMENDED READING

Baldwin CJ, Ledet AE: Pancytopenia. In August JR, editor: *Consultations in feline medicine,* Philadelphia, 1994, WB Saunders.

Jordan HL, Grindem CB, Breitschwerdt EB: Thrombocytopenia in cats: a retrospective study of 41 cases, *J Vet Internal Med* 7:261, 1993.

PROBLEM 28 Answer Key

1. 0	22. 0	42. +
2. 0	23. +	43. –
3. +	24. +	44. 0
4. +	25. 0	45. –
5. +	26. 0	46. –
6. +	27. 0	47. –
7. 0	28. 0	48. –
8. 0	29. +	49. –
9. +	30. +	50. –
10. +	31. +	51. –
11. 0	32. +	52. –
12. 0	33. +	53. –
13. 0	34. +	54. –
14. 0	35. +	55. +
15. 0	36. +	56. –
16. 0	37. 0	57. –
17. +	38. 0	58. –
18. 0	39. +	59. –
19. 0	40. +	60. +
20. +	41. 0	61. –
21. +		

+ = clearly indicated   – = contraindicated   0 = neutral

Total Positive Responses _____

Total Neutral Responses _____

Total Negative Responses _____

RECOMMENDED READING

DiBartola SP et al: Clinicopathologic findings resembling hypoadrenocorticism in dogs with primary gastrointestinal disease, *JAVMA* 187:60, 1985.

PROBLEM 29 Answer Key

1. +	22. +	43. 0
2. +	23. 0	44. −
3. +	24. 0	45. +
4. +	25. 0	46. +
5. 0	26. 0	47. −
6. +	27. 0	48. −
7. +	28. +	49. +
8. 0	29. 0	50. −
9. 0	30. 0	51. +
10. 0	31. 0	52. +
11. 0	32. +	53. +
12. +	33. 0	54. +
13. 0	34. 0	55. −
14. 0	35. +	56. −
15. 0	36. 0	57. −
16. 0	37. +	58. −
17. 0	38. +	59. −
18. 0	39. +	60. −
19. 0	40. 0	61. −
20. +	41. −	62. −
21. +	42. +	63. +

+ = clearly indicated − = contraindicated 0 = neutral

Total Positive Responses _____

Total Neutral Responses _____

Total Negative Responses _____

RECOMMENDED READING

Bunch SE: Hepatobiliary and exocrine pancreatic disorders. In Nelson RW, Couto CG, editors: *Essentials of small animal medicine,* St. Louis, 1992, Mosby.

Center SA: Feline liver disorders and their management, *Comp Cont Educ* 8:889, 1986.

Jacobs et al: Treatment of idiopathic hepatic lipidosis in cats: 11 cases (1986-1987), *JAVMA* 195:635, 1989.

PROBLEM 30 Answer Key

1. +	22. 0	43. +
2. 0	23. +	44. +
3. 0	24. 0	45. −
4. +	25. 0	46. −
5. 0	26. 0	47. −
6. +	27. 0	48. −
7. +	28. 0	49. −
8. 0	29. 0	50. −
9. 0	30. +	51. +
10. +	31. +	52. 0
11. +	32. 0	53. −
12. 0	33. 0	54. −
13. 0	34. 0	55. 0
14. 0	35. +	56. −
15. 0	36. +	57. −
16. 0	37. 0	58. −
17. +	38. 0	59. −
18. +	39. 0	60. +
19. +	40. 0	61. −
20. +	41. −	62. −
21. +	42. 0	

+ = clearly indicated − = contraindicated 0 = neutral

Total Positive Responses _____

Total Neutral Responses _____

Total Negative Responses _____

RECOMMENDED READING

Orton EC: Gastric dilatation volvulus. In Kirk RW, editor: *Current veterinary therapy IX,* Philadelphia, 1985, WB Saunders.

Strombeck DR, Guilford WG: Gastric dilatation volvulus. In Strombeck DR, Guilford WG, editors: *Small animal gastroenterology,* ed 2, Davis, Calif., 1990, Stonegate.

Twedt DC, Magne ML: Diseases of the stomach. In Ettinger SJ, editor: *Textbook of veterinary internal medicine,* ed 3, Philadelphia, 1989, WB Saunders.

PROBLEM 31 Answer Key

1. +	20. 0	39. 0
2. +	21. 0	40. 0
3. 0	22. +	41. −
4. +	23. 0	42. +
5. 0	24. 0	43. 0
6. +	25. +	44. +
7. +	26. 0	45. +
8. +	27. 0	46. −
9. +	28. 0	47. −
10. 0	29. 0	48. −
11. 0	30. +	49. −
12. 0	31. 0	50. −
13. +	32. 0	51. −
14. 0	33. 0	52. −
15. 0	34. 0	53. −
16. 0	35. 0	54. −
17. 0	36. +	55. +
18. 0	37. +	56. −
19. 0	38. 0	57. −

+ = clearly indicated   − = contraindicated   0 = neutral

Total Positive Responses _____

Total Neutral Responses _____

Total Negative Responses _____

RECOMMENDED READING

Kruger JM et al: Clinical evaluation of cats with lower urinary tract disease, *JAVMA* 199:211, 1991.

Osorne CA et al: Feline lower urinary tract disorders. In Ettinger SJ, editor: *Textbook of veterinary internal medicine,* ed 3, Philadelphia, 1989, WB Saunders.

PROBLEM 32 Answer Key

1. +	22. +	43. −
2. +	23. 0	44. 0
3. 0	24. +	45. −
4. 0	25. 0	46. −
5. 0	26. 0	47. −
6. +	27. +	48. −
7. +	28. 0	49. −
8. 0	29. 0	50. −
9. +	30. +	51. −
10. +	31. +	52. −
11. +	32. +	53. −
12. 0	33. 0	54. −
13. 0	34. +	55. +
14. +	35. 0	56. −
15. 0	36. 0	57. +
16. +	37. +	58. −
17. +	38. −	59. −
18. +	39. +	60. −
19. +	40. 0	61. −
20. +	41. −	62. −
21. +	42. 0	

+ = clearly indicated   − = contraindicated   0 = neutral

Total Positive Responses _____

Total Neutral Responses _____

Total Negative Responses _____

RECOMMENDED READING

Feldman EC, Nelson RW: Canine female reproduction. In Feldman EC, Nelson RW, editors: *Canine and feline endocrinology and reproduction,* ed 2, Philadelphia, 1996, WB Saunders.

Feldman EC, Nelson RW: Diagnostic and therapeutic alternatives for pyometra in dogs and cats. In Kirk RW, editor: *Current veterinary therapy X,* Philadelphia, 1989, WB Saunders.

PROBLEM 33 Answer Key

1. +	20. +	38. −
2. +	21. +	39. 0
3. 0	22. 0	40. 0
4. +	23. 0	41. −
5. 0	24. 0	42. 0
6. 0	25. 0	43. −
7. 0	26. 0	44. +
8. +	27. 0	45. −
9. 0	28. +	46. −
10. 0	29. 0	47. −
11. 0	30. 0	48. +
12. 0	31. 0	49. −
13. 0	32. 0	50. −
14. 0	33. 0	51. −
15. 0	34. 0	52. −
16. 0	35. +	53. +
17. 0	36. +	54. −
18. 0	37. +	55. −
19. 0		

+ = clearly indicated   − = contraindicated   0 = neutral

Total Positive Responses _____

Total Neutral Responses _____

Total Negative Responses _____

RECOMMENDED READING

Birchard S, Carothers M: Aggressive surgery for the management of oral neoplasia, *Vet Clin North Am* 20:1117, 1989.
Cotter SM: Oral pharyngeal neoplasms in the cat, *J Am Animal Hosp Assoc* 17:917, 1981.

PROBLEM 34 Answer Key

1. +	22. 0	43. +
2. +	23. 0	44. −
3. +	24. 0	45. −
4. +	25. 0	46. 0
5. 0	26. 0	47. −
6. +	27. +	48. −
7. +	28. +	49. −
8. +	29. +	50. −
9. +	30. +	51. −
10. +	31. 0	52. −
11. 0	32. 0	53. −
12. 0	33. 0	54. −
13. +	34. 0	55. −
14. 0	35. 0	56. −
15. 0	36. −	57. −
16. +	37. 0	58. −
17. 0	38. −	59. −
18. 0	39. −	60. −
19. 0	40. +	61. −
20. 0	41. +	62. +
21. 0	42. −	

+ = clearly indicated   − = contraindicated   0 = neutral

Total Positive Responses _____

Total Neutral Responses _____

Total Negative Responses _____

RECOMMENDED READING

Lenehan TM et al: Canine panosteitis. In Newton CD, Nunamaker DM, editors: *Textbook of small animal orthopedics,* Philadelphia, 1985, Lippincott.

PROBLEM 35 Answer Key

1. +	19. 0	37. +
2. +	20. +	38. +
3. 0	21. 0	39. +
4. +	22. 0	40. +
5. 0	23. 0	41. −
6. 0	24. 0	42. −
7. 0	25. +	43. 0
8. +	26. 0	44. +
9. 0	27. 0	45. 0
10. 0	28. +	46. −
11. 0	29. +	47. −
12. 0	30. 0	48. −
13. +	31. +	49. −
14. +	32. 0	50. −
15. 0	33. 0	51. −
16. 0	34. 0	52. +
17. 0	35. 0	53. −
18. 0	36. 0	

+ = clearly indicated   − = contraindicated   0 = neutral

Total Positive Responses _____

Total Neutral Responses _____

Total Negative Responses _____

RECOMMENDED READING

Couto CG: Disorders of hemostasis. In Nelson RW, Couto CG, editors: *Essentials of small animal internal medicine,* St. Louis, 1992, Mosby.

Mount ME: Diagnosis and therapy of anticoagulant rodenticide intoxication, *Vet Clin North Am* 18:115, 1988.

PROBLEM 36 Answer Key

1. +	22. 0	42. −
2. +	23. 0	43. −
3. +	24. 0	44. +
4. +	25. 0	45. +
5. 0	26. 0	46. 0
6. 0	27. +	47. −
7. 0	28. 0	48. −
8. 0	29. 0	49. +
9. +	30. 0	50. +
10. +	31. +	51. −
11. 0	32. 0	52. −
12. +	33. +	53. 0
13. +	34. −	54. 0
14. +	35. 0	55. 0
15. 0	36. +	56. −
16. 0	37. 0	57. +
17. 0	38. 0	58. −
18. 0	39. 0	59. −
19. 0	40. +	60. −
20. 0	41. +	61. −
21. 0		

+ = clearly indicated   − = contraindicated   0 = neutral

Total Positive Responses _____

Total Neutral Responses _____

Total Negative Responses _____

RECOMMENDED READING

Caywood DD et al: Pancreatic insulin-secreting neoplasms: Clinical, diagnostic, and prognostic features in 73 dogs, *J Am An Hosp Assoc* 24:577, 1988.

Feldman EC, Nelson RW: Hypoglycemia. In Feldman EC, Nelson RW, editors: *Canine and feline endocrinology and reproduction,* Philadelphia, 1987, WB Saunders.

PROBLEM 37 Answer Key

1. +	22. 0	42. +
2. +	23. 0	43. 0
3. +	24. 0	44. +
4. +	25. 0	45. −
5. +	26. 0	46. +
6. +	27. +	47. −
7. +	28. 0	48. +
8. +	29. 0	49. −
9. +	30. 0	50. −
10. +	31. 0	51. 0
11. 0	32. 0	52. 0
12. 0	33. 0	53. +
13. 0	34. +	54. −
14. 0	35. +	55. −
15. 0	36. 0	56. −
16. 0	37. +	57. −
17. 0	38. +	58. −
18. 0	39. +	59. −
19. 0	40. −	60. −
20. 0	41. +	61. +
21. +		

+ = clearly indicated   − = contraindicated   0 = neutral

Total Positive Responses _____

Total Neutral Responses _____

Total Negative Responses _____

RECOMMENDED READING

Dennis JS et al: Lymphocytic/plasmacytic gastroenteritis in cats: 14 cases (1985-1990), *J Am Vet Med Assoc* 200:1712, 1992.

Willard MD: Inflammatory bowel disease: perspectives on therapy, *J Am An Hosp Assoc* 28:27, 1992.

PROBLEM 38 Answer Key

1. 0	22. +	43. +
2. +	23. +	44. 0
3. 0	24. 0	45. 0
4. +	25. 0	46. 0
5. 0	26. 0	47. +
6. 0	27. 0	48. +
7. +	28. 0	49. −
8. 0	29. +	50. +
9. +	30. +	51. −
10. +	31. +	52. −
11. 0	32. +	53. 0
12. 0	33. 0	54. +
13. 0	34. 0	55. 0
14. 0	35. +	56. −
15. +	36. +	57. −
16. 0	37. 0	58. −
17. 0	38. 0	59. +
18. 0	39. +	60. −
19. 0	40. +	61. −
20. 0	41. −	62. −
21. 0	42. +	

+ = clearly indicated   − = contraindicated   0 = neutral

Total Positive Responses _____

Total Neutral Responses _____

Total Negative Responses _____

RECOMMENDED READING

Johnson SE: Canine eosinophilic gastroenterocolitis, *Sem Vet Med Surg (SA)* 7:145, 1992.

Willard MD: Disorders of the intestinal tract. In Nelson RW, Couto CG, editors: *Essentials of small animal internal medicine,* St. Louis, 1992, Mosby.

PROBLEM 39 Answer Key

1. +	22. 0	42. +
2. +	23. 0	43. −
3. +	24. 0	44. +
4. 0	25. 0	45. +
5. 0	26. +	46. +
6. 0	27. +	47. 0
7. +	28. 0	48. +
8. 0	29. 0	49. 0
9. +	30. 0	50. 0
10. 0	31. 0	51. −
11. 0	32. 0	52. −
12. +	33. 0	53. +
13. 0	34. 0	54. +
14. 0	35. 0	55. −
15. 0	36. −	56. −
16. 0	37. +	57. +
17. 0	38. +	58. −
18. 0	39. +	59. −
19. 0	40. +	60. −
20. +	41. +	61. −
21. 0		

+ = clearly indicated   − = contraindicated   0 = neutral

Total Positive Responses _____

Total Neutral Responses _____

Total Negative Responses _____

RECOMMENDED READING

Dubey JP, Carpenter JL: Histologically confirmed clinical
   toxoplasmosis in cats: 100 cases (1952-1990), *J Am Vet Med
   Assoc* 203:1556, 1993.
Lappin MR et al: Enzyme-linked immunosorbent assays for the
   detection of *Toxoplasma gondii*—specific antibodies and antigens
   in the aqueous humor of cats, *J Am Vet Med Assoc* 201:1010,
   1992.

PROBLEM 40 Answer Key

1. +	22. 0	43. +
2. +	23. 0	44. +
3. 0	24. 0	45. 0
4. 0	25. 0	46. −
5. +	26. 0	47. −
6. 0	27. 0	48. −
7. 0	28. 0	49. +
8. +	29. +	50. −
9. +	30. +	51. 0
10. 0	31. 0	52. −
11. 0	32. 0	53. 0
12. +	33. +	54. −
13. +	34. 0	55. −
14. +	35. +	56. −
15. 0	36. +	57. −
16. 0	37. 0	58. −
17. +	38. 0	59. +
18. +	39. +	60. −
19. +	40. +	61. −
20. +	41. +	62. −
21. +	42. +	63. −

+ = clearly indicated   − = contraindicated   0 = neutral

Total Positive Responses _____

Total Neutral Responses _____

Total Negative Responses _____

RECOMMENDED READING

Campbell KL: Diagnosis and management of polycythemia in dogs,
   Comp Cont Educ 12:543, 1990.
Peterson ME, Randolf JF: Diagnosis and treatment of polycythemia. In
   Kirk RW, editor: *Current veterinary therapy VIII,* Philadelphia,
   1983, WB Saunders.

PROBLEM 41 Answer Key

1. +	22. +	43. +
2. +	23. 0	44. 0
3. +	24. 0	45. −
4. +	25. +	46. −
5. 0	26. 0	47. −
6. +	27. 0	48. −
7. +	28. +	49. 0
8. 0	29. +	50. −
9. 0	30. +	51. −
10. +	31. +	52. +
11. +	32. 0	53. −
12. +	33. 0	54. +
13. 0	34. +	55. −
14. 0	35. 0	56. −
15. +	36. −	57. −
16. +	37. +	58. −
17. 0	38. 0	59. −
18. 0	39. 0	60. −
19. 0	40. 0	61. −
20. +	41. −	62. −
21. 0	42. +	63. +

+ = clearly indicated   − = contraindicated   0 = neutral

Total Positive Responses _____

Total Neutral Responses _____

Total Negative Responses _____

RECOMMENDED READING

Basher AWP, Fowler JD: Conservative versus surgical management of gastrointestinal linear foreign bodies in the cat, *Vet Surg* 16:135, 1987.

Felts JF et al: Thread and sewing needle as gastrointestinal foreign bodies in the cat: a review of 64 cases, *J Am Vet Med Assoc* 184:56, 1984.

PROBLEM 42 Answer Key

1. +	23. +	44. +
2. 0	24. 0	45. +
3. +	25. 0	46. −
4. +	26. 0	47. 0
5. +	27. 0	48. −
6. +	28. 0	49. −
7. +	29. +	50. 0
8. 0	30. +	51. +
9. +	31. +	52. 0
10. +	32. +	53. −
11. +	33. 0	54. +
12. +	34. 0	55. 0
13. 0	35. −	56. −
14. 0	36. 0	57. −
15. 0	37. 0	58. 0
16. +	38. 0	59. −
17. +	39. 0	60. +
18. +	40. +	61. −
19. +	41. −	62. −
20. +	42. +	63. −
21. +	43. +	64. −
22. 0		

+ = clearly indicated   − = contraindicated   0 = neutral

Total Positive Responses _____

Total Neutral Responses _____

Total Negative Responses _____

RECOMMENDED READING

Klag AR et al: Idiopathic immune-mediated hemolytic anemia in dogs: 42 cases (1986-1990), *J Am Vet Med Assoc* 202:783, 1993.

Stewart AF, Feldman BF: Immune-mediated hemolytic anemia. Part II. Clinical entity, diagnosis, and treatment theory, *Comp Cont Educ* 15:1479, 1993.

PROBLEM 43 Answer Key

1. +	23. 0	44. 0
2. 0	24. +	45. +
3. +	25. 0	46. –
4. +	26. +	47. 0
5. +	27. 0	48. 0
6. +	28. 0	49. 0
7. 0	29. 0	50. 0
8. 0	30. +	51. 0
9. 0	31. 0	52. 0
10. +	32. 0	53. –
11. +	33. 0	54. –
12. +	34. 0	55. 0
13. 0	35. –	56. 0
14. 0	36. 0	57. +
15. +	37. 0	58. –
16. 0	38. +	59. –
17. 0	39. 0	60. –
18. 0	40. 0	61. –
19. 0	41. –	62. +
20. 0	42. +	63. –
21. 0	43. +	64. –
22. 0		

+ = clearly indicated   – = contraindicated   0 = neutral

Total Positive Responses _____

Total Neutral Responses _____

Total Negative Responses _____

RECOMMENDED READING

Feldman EC, Nelson RW: Canine hypothyroidism. In Feldman EC, Nelson RW, editors: *Canine and feline endocrinology and reproduction,* ed 2, Philadelphia, 1996, WB Saunders.

Panciera DL: Canine hypothyroidism. Part I. Clinical findings and control of thyroid hormone secretion and metabolism, *Comp Cont Educ* 12:689, 1990.

Panciera DL: Canine hypothyroidism. Part II. Thyroid function tests and treatment, *Comp Cont Educ* 12:843, 1990.